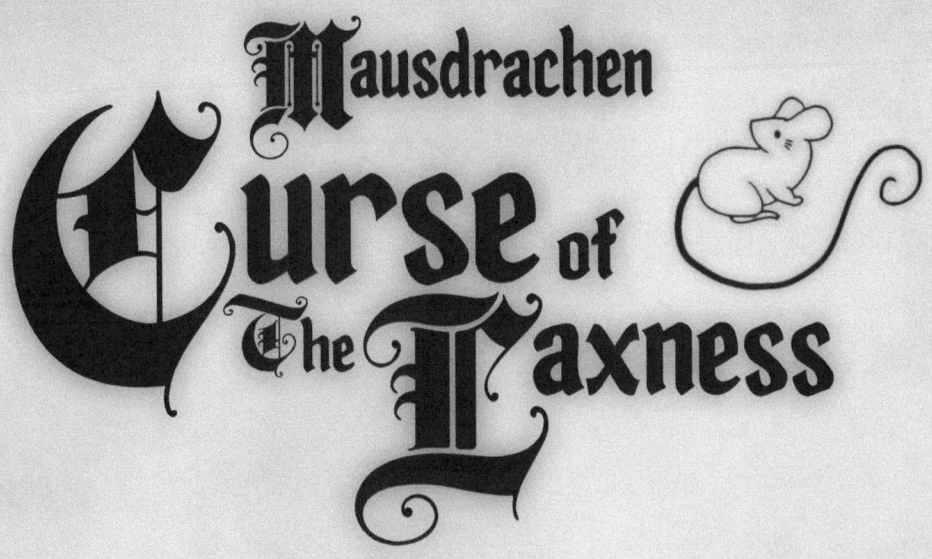

Mausdrachen Curse of The Taxness

written by
Thea Kvamme

illustrated by
Samantha Hinton

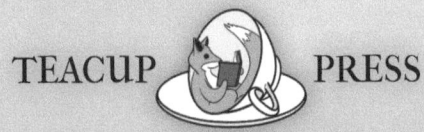

TEACUP PRESS

To my mom:
what the mind forgets,
the heart will always remember

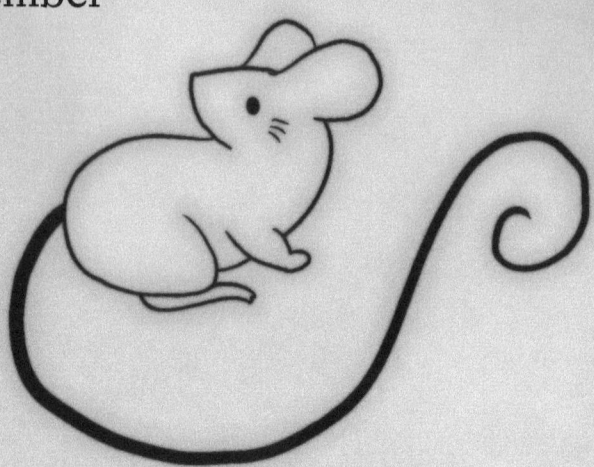

www.teacup-press.com
www.foxpointepublishing.com/author-thea-kvamme

Library of Congress Cataloging-in-Publication Data
Kvamme, Thea, author.
Hinton, Samantha, illustrator.
Farr, Chelsea, editor & designer.
Mausdrachen: Curse of The Laxness / Thea Kvamme. – First edition.
Summary: A mother and daughter go on a quest with a mouse-dragon to rescue a grandmother from a memory curse.
ISBN 979-8-9938504-0-5 (hardcover) / 979-8-9938504-1-2 (softcover)
[1. Fairy tales. 2. Dragons – Fiction. 3. Mice – Fiction. 4. Disease – Fiction. 5. Family – Fiction.]
Library of Congress Control Number: 2 0 2 0 9 0 8 2 3 7

Second printing January 2026

a Note from the Author

Alzheimer's Disease is something many people will encounter in their lifetimes. Children can have an especially hard time understanding why their grandparent keeps forgetting things or repeating themselves.

Always remind your children that their grandparent or other family member is still the same person deep down, and they will still love them no matter what.

It is my hope that this book will help children understand what happens with Alzheimer's Disease, and when needed, give them a little break in a make-believe world.

Thank you for reading *Mausdrachen: Curse of The Laxness*.

-Thea Kvamme

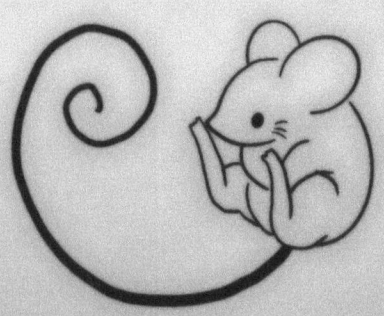

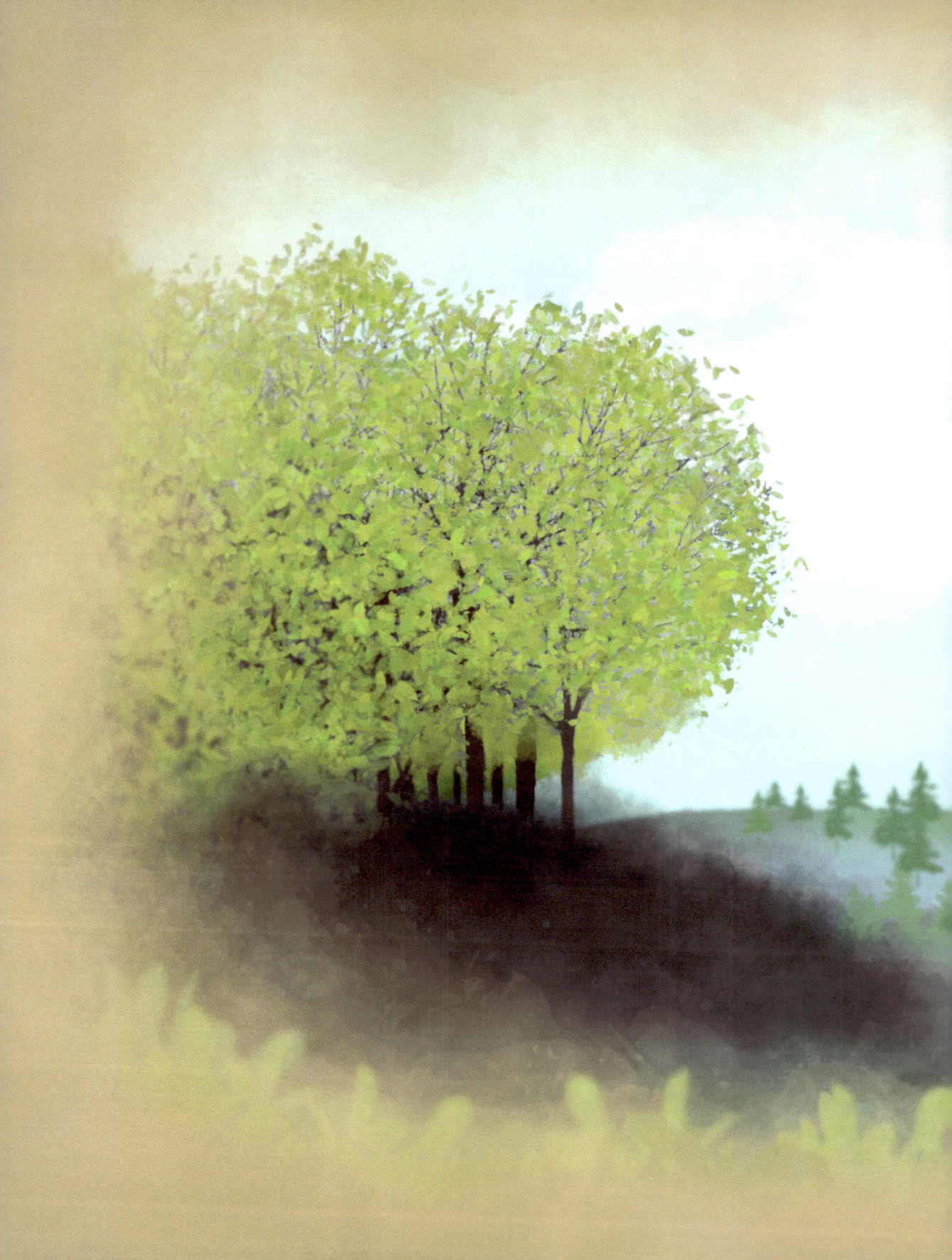

The Laxness was known for breaking hearts.
It crept. It stole. It slithered and consumed.
You wouldn't see it coming.
It especially loved memories.

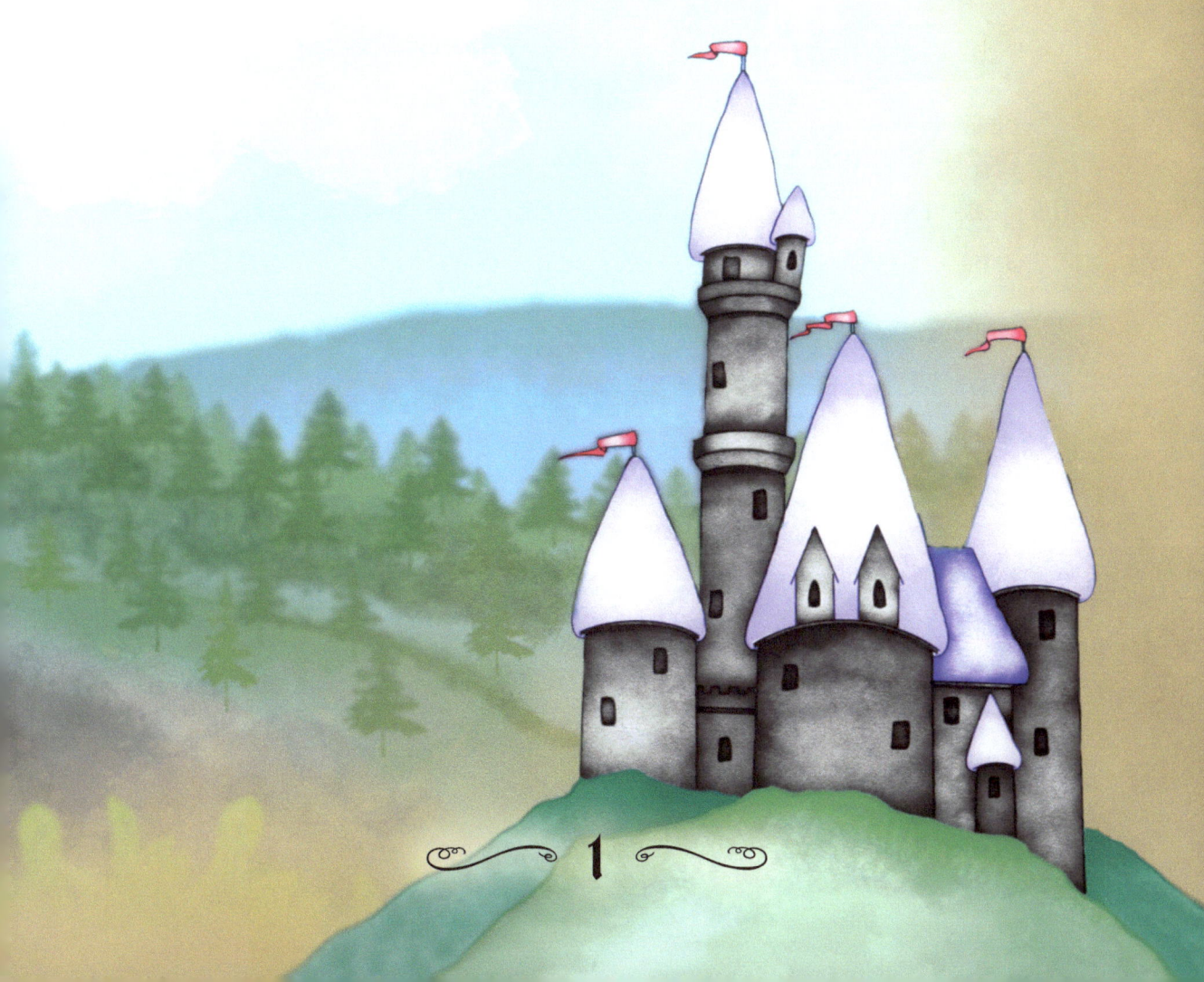

Chapter One

It was a beautiful day and Queen Dorothy of Engelmaus had decided to go pick some flowers for her daughter, Elaine, and granddaughter, Hannah. She walked out of the gates of the castle toward the Forest of Flowers. It was the perfect time for flowers, as they were in full bloom.

The Queen walked into the forest and noticed how wonderful the flowers looked today. She started to pick the ones she knew Elaine and Hannah would love: pink, white, yellow . . .

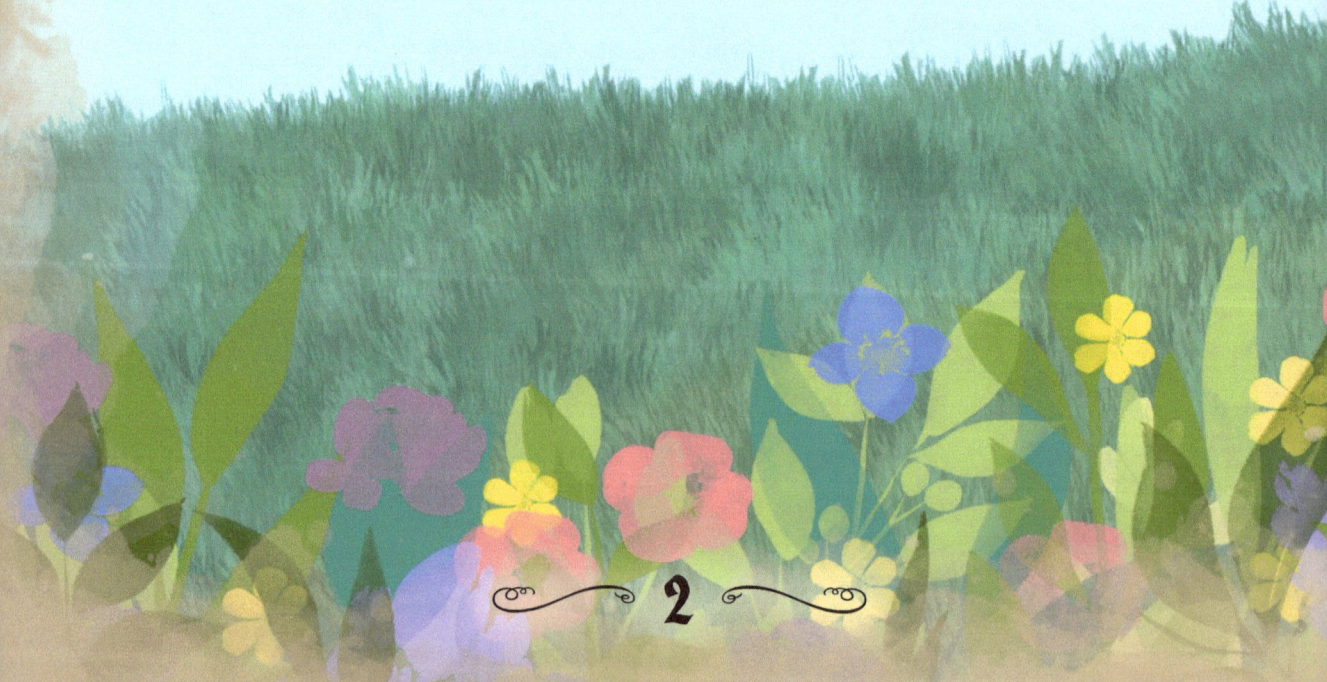

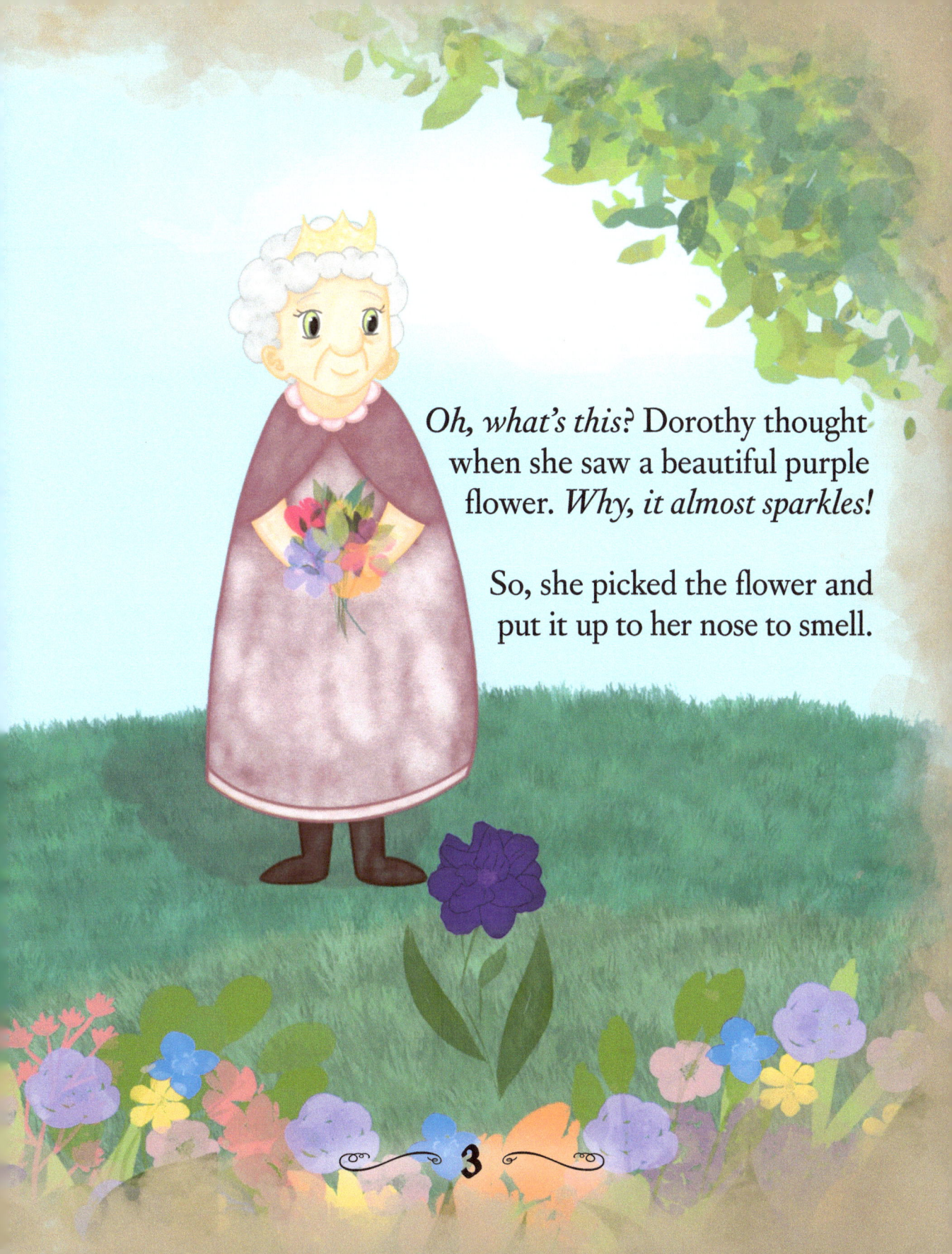

Oh, what's this? Dorothy thought when she saw a beautiful purple flower. *Why, it almost sparkles!*

So, she picked the flower and put it up to her nose to smell.

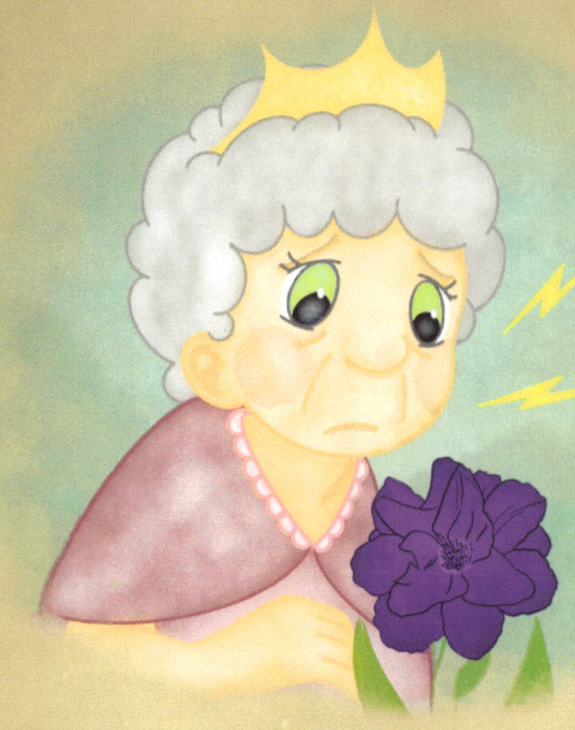

OUCH! She thought a bee had stung her, but she didn't see any bees.

OUCH! She felt a new zap, but this time on her nose – she looked around and didn't recognize where she was. The flower didn't look as pretty now. It started to look dark and withered, and it was still zapping her.

She tried to let go, but the flower stem had wrapped tightly around her wrist. No matter what she did, there was no escape. She thought of her granddaughter playing nearby and began to yell for help, "Hannah! Hannah, can you hear me?"

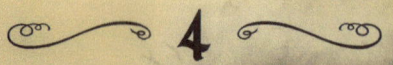

A gray fog came over Dorothy then and she couldn't see where she was or how to get out. She was scared. She felt like she was forgetting things now.

It's so hard to remember anything with all of this fog. I just want to go home... Why is it getting dark so fast?

She started to shake with fear, yelling, "Hannah! Please, please help me!"

Why did I come out here in the first place? Where was I going? Am I forgetting things or am I just scared?

Queen Dorothy started to cry.

I'm lost.

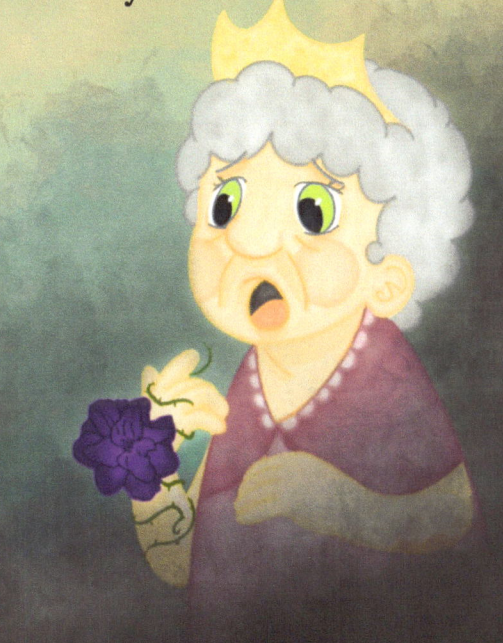

Chapter Two

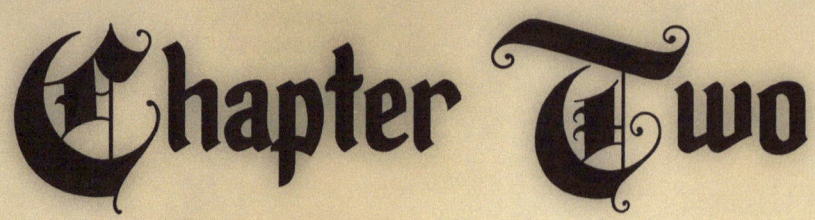

Princess Hannah and Mausdrachen were playing outside that day on the grassy hills near the Forest of Flowers. Mausdrachen was Hannah's closest friend. She had known him for years and she still called him "Mausy," something she'd first started doing when she was just learning to speak and couldn't pronounce Mausdrachen's name yet.

Mausdrachen was a magnificent creature. He had soft gray fur with big round ears, a stubby little nose, and beautiful pink wings that sparkled in the light. He also had a long tail that Hannah would use to climb up on his back so they could go flying together.

Today was being spent flying kites instead and watching the clouds in the sky. Hannah always enjoyed telling Mausdrachen what she saw while looking at the clouds.

"Mausy, do you see that fish?" Hannah asked, pointing at a lumpy white cloud.

Mausdrachen twitched his nose in response. He enjoyed looking at the clouds with Hannah, but he liked flying through them even better.

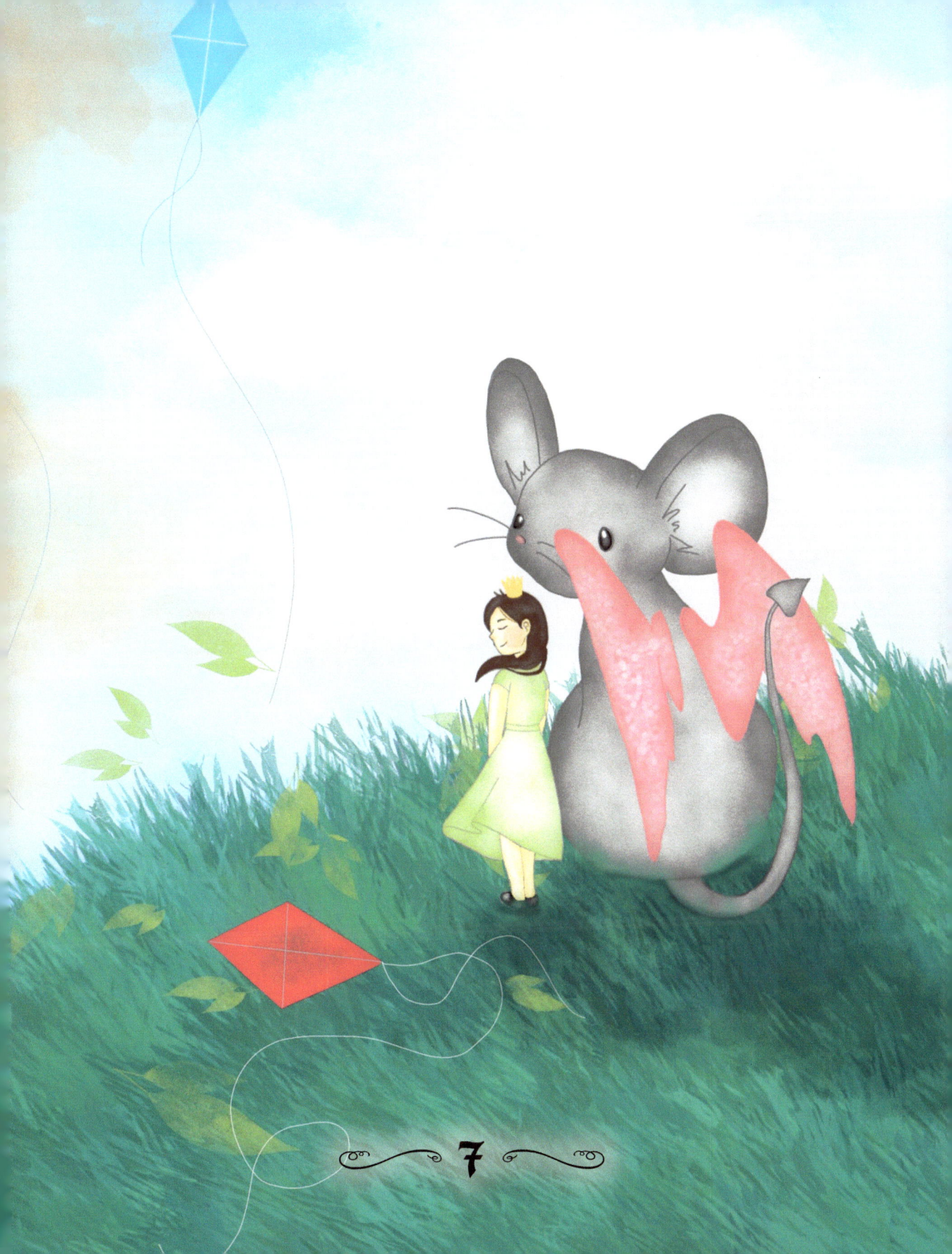

All of a sudden, Mausdrachen's ears perked up.

"What's wrong?" Hannah asked.

Mausdrachen sat still, listening. Faintly, Hannah heard someone yell for help. Beside her, Mausdrachen's nose twitched again. He sniffed the air, confused.

Hannah heard a voice call: "Hannah, please help me!" It was so distant she could barely understand the words.

Is that Grandma? Where would she be? Is she okay? Hannah wondered, growing worried.

Mausdrachen gave Hannah a nudge and she quickly climbed on his back and held onto the fur on his neck, ready to fly.

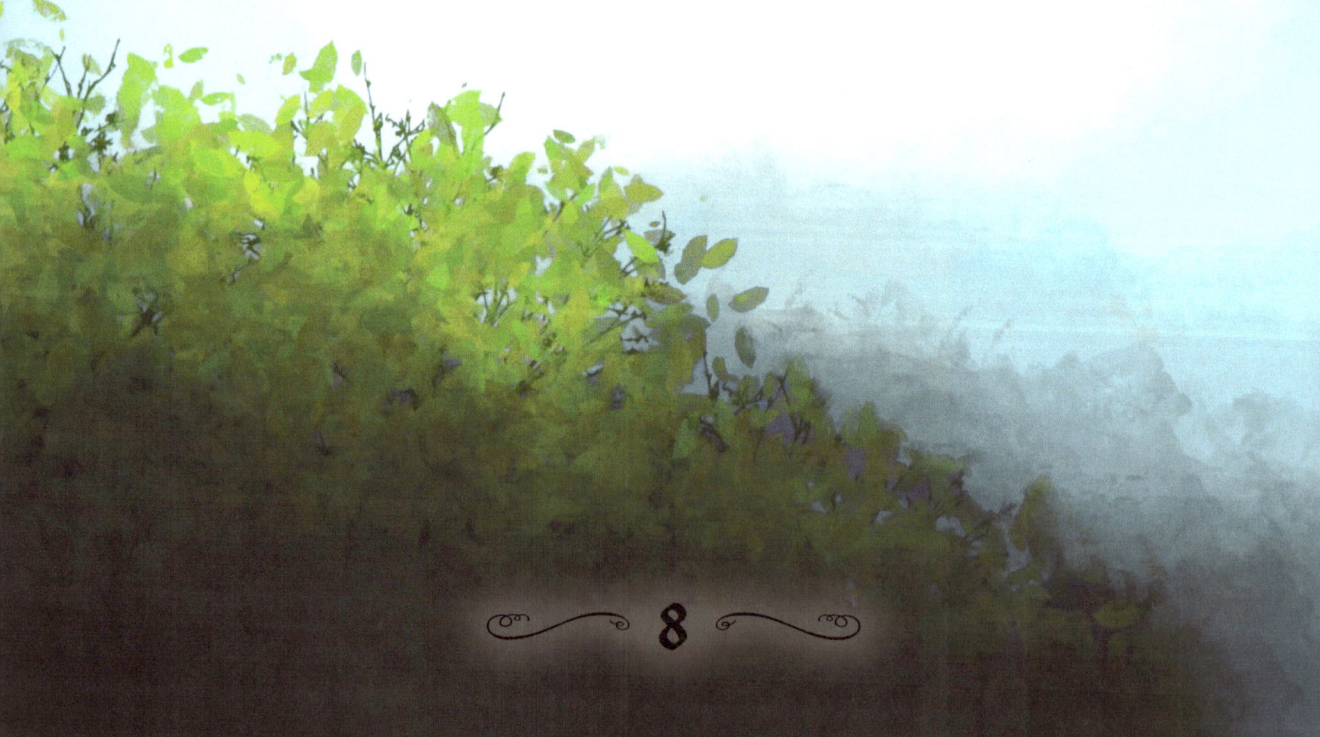

As they flew toward the castle, they noticed a gray fog in the distance. *What is that? I've never seen it before!* Hannah thought to herself.

They flew closer to see if they could get a better look. The fog was swirling and churning in on itself. It was taking over the Forest of Flowers. Hannah thought, *I don't know what it is, but I can't see into it at all!* Mausdrachen seemed hesitant to get any closer.

"I know! I'm scared too, Mausy!" Hannah yelled over the sound of the air rushing past them.

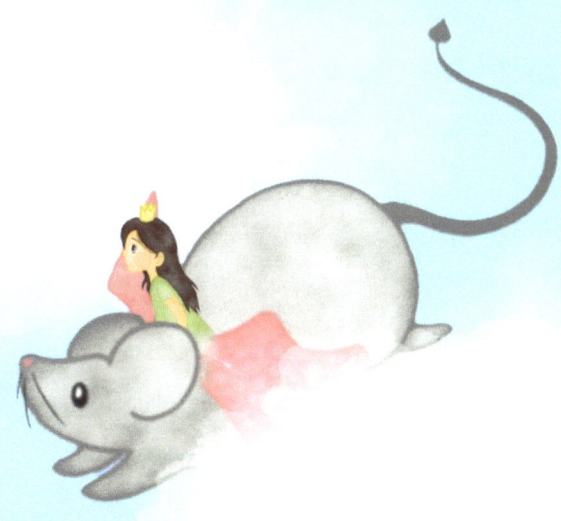

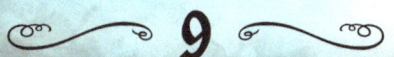

"Help! Someone please save me!"

This time, they were both able to hear Queen Dorothy's call for help clearly. But all Hannah and Mausdrachen could see was the fog and it was growing rapidly, draining the color from the world around it as it spread. They watched trails of light swirling through the sky until they collided with the fog cloud and vanished.

"Grandma? Grandma, are you there?" Hannah cried out. She waited a moment but didn't hear Queen Dorothy again. She held onto Mausdrachen tighter, feeling scared and worried.

"Oh Mausy, I can't see anything in there! We need to get help! Let's get back to the castle!"

Mausdrachen swung around in the sky, turning them back towards home.

"Mausy, I know Grandma is in that fog back there. We have to find her."

Chapter Three

Mausdrachen landed near the castle's entrance and Hannah immediately jumped off his back, running into the castle to find help. She soon found Princess Elaine, her mother.

"Mama! I heard Grandma calling for help but I can't find her! Will you come help me?"

"Of course I will, Hannah. Where did you hear her?"

"It sounds like she's in the Forest of Flowers, but there's a thick fog surrounding it and I can't see anything!"

"Alright, we'll go look for her together. Go wait outside with Mausdrachen," Elaine instructed. "I have to see if Grandma took her amulet with her today."

"Her amulet? What's that?"

"It's the heart-shaped necklace she always wears. She said it helps remind her of special times whenever she feels lost," Elaine explained. "If she forgot to wear it today, maybe that's why she's lost in the Forest of Flowers."

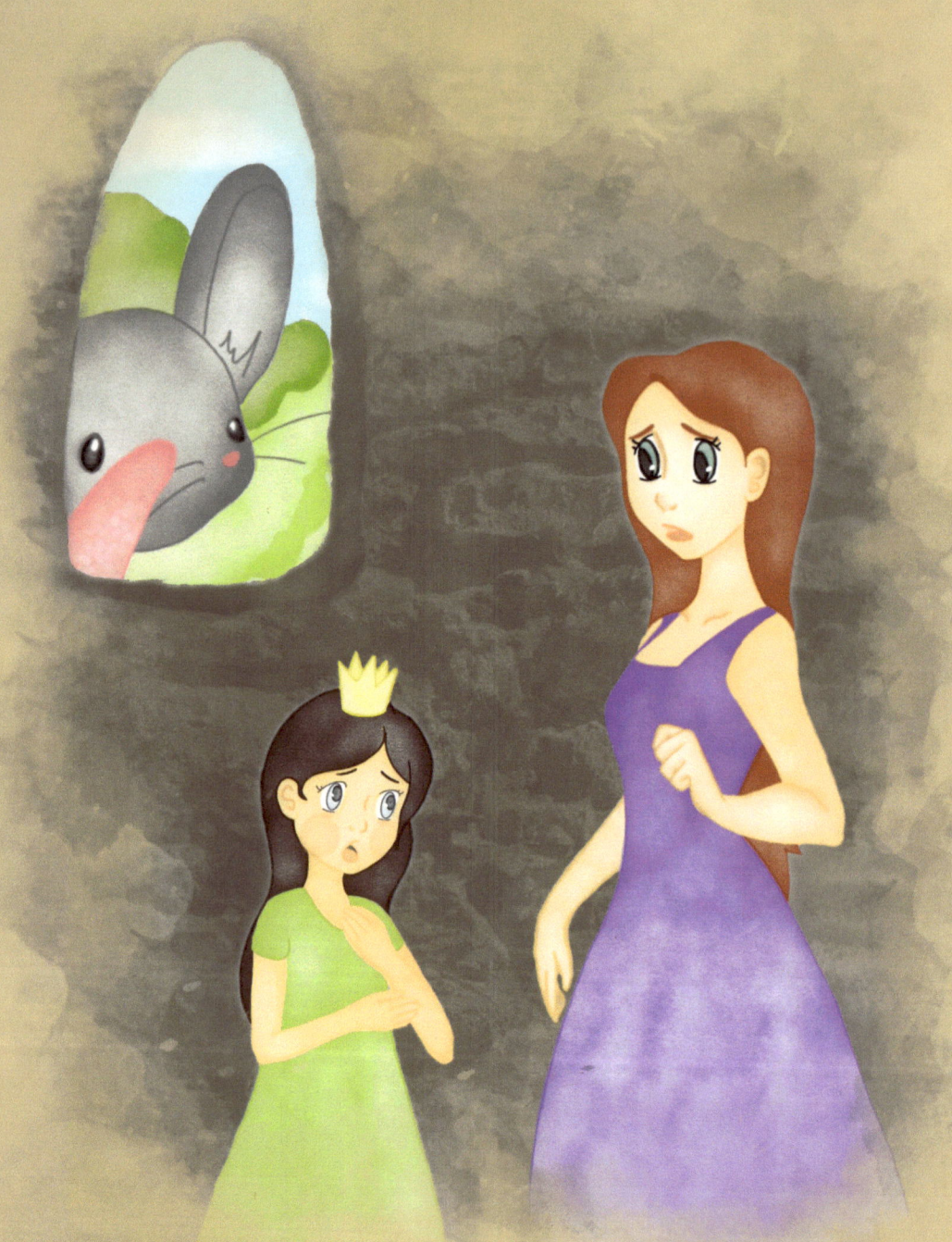

Elaine ran up the stairs to Queen Dorothy's room while Hannah went back out to Mausdrachen. When Elaine got to her mother's room, she saw the amulet hanging on the mirror.

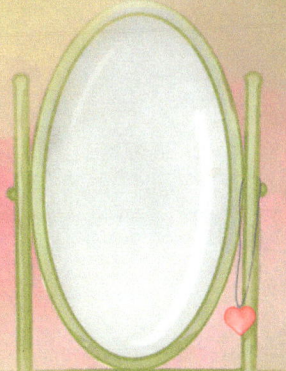

Oh no! I was right! We have to get this to her!

Elaine grabbed the dangling pendant and ran outside where Hannah and Mausdrachen were waiting. The young princess was already perched on Mausdrachen's back.

"Did you find Grandma's amulet?" Hannah asked.

Nodding, Elaine opened her hand and showed Hannah the heart-shaped amulet – it wasn't as pretty as Hannah remembered. It looked faded and dull.

"Hannah, would you wear it until we find Grandma? I don't want it to get lost," Elaine said.

"Yes!"

Elaine quickly climbed up on Mausdrachen's back, then fastened the amulet on Hannah's neck.

"Let's go!" they both told Mausdrachen. With that, he leapt into the sky.

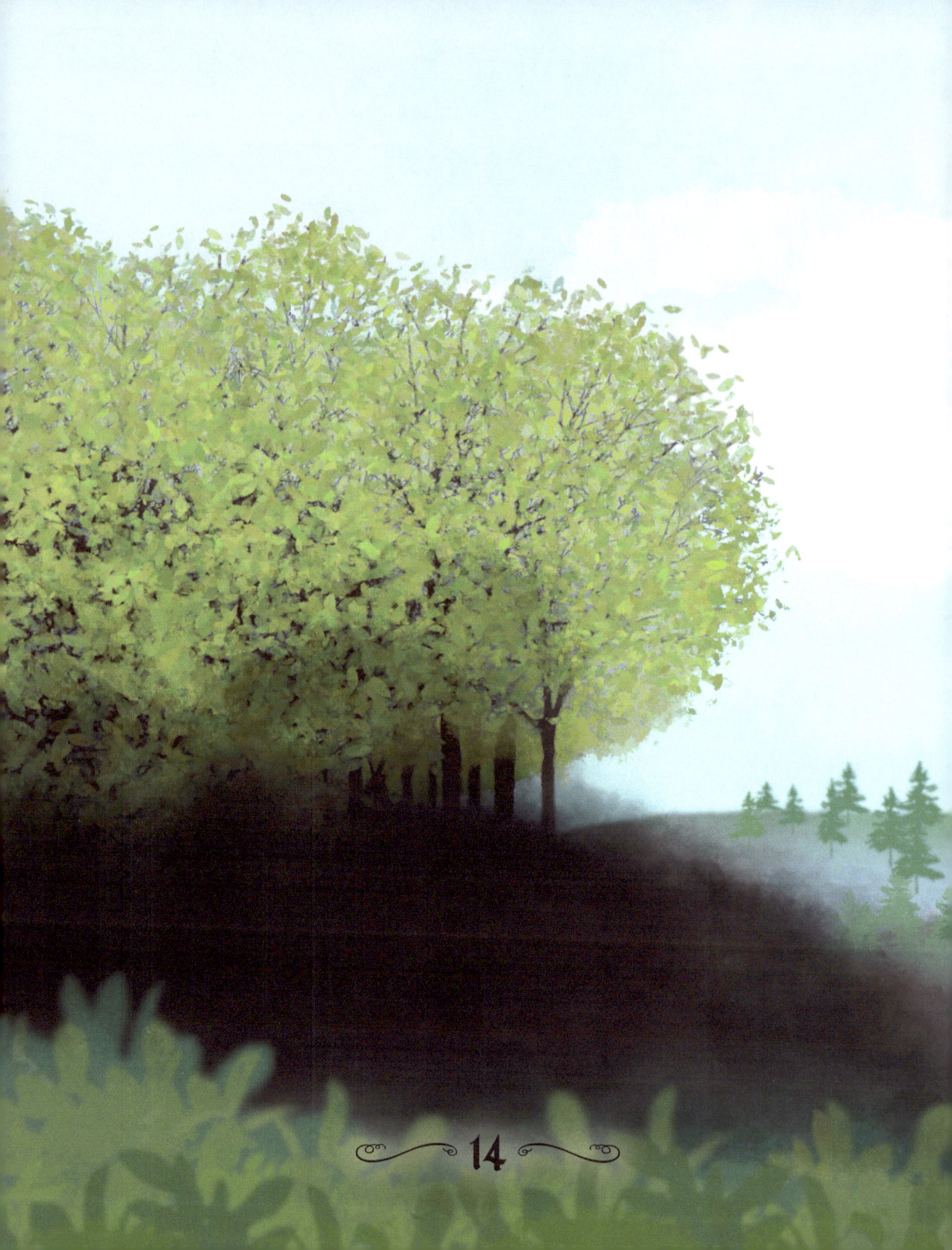

14

Mausdrachen flew towards the Forest of Flowers. Hannah could see the fog had grown even bigger while they were at the castle. The closer Mausdrachen flew to the Forest, the more terrified Hannah felt. *If Grandma is in there, she must be so scared!*

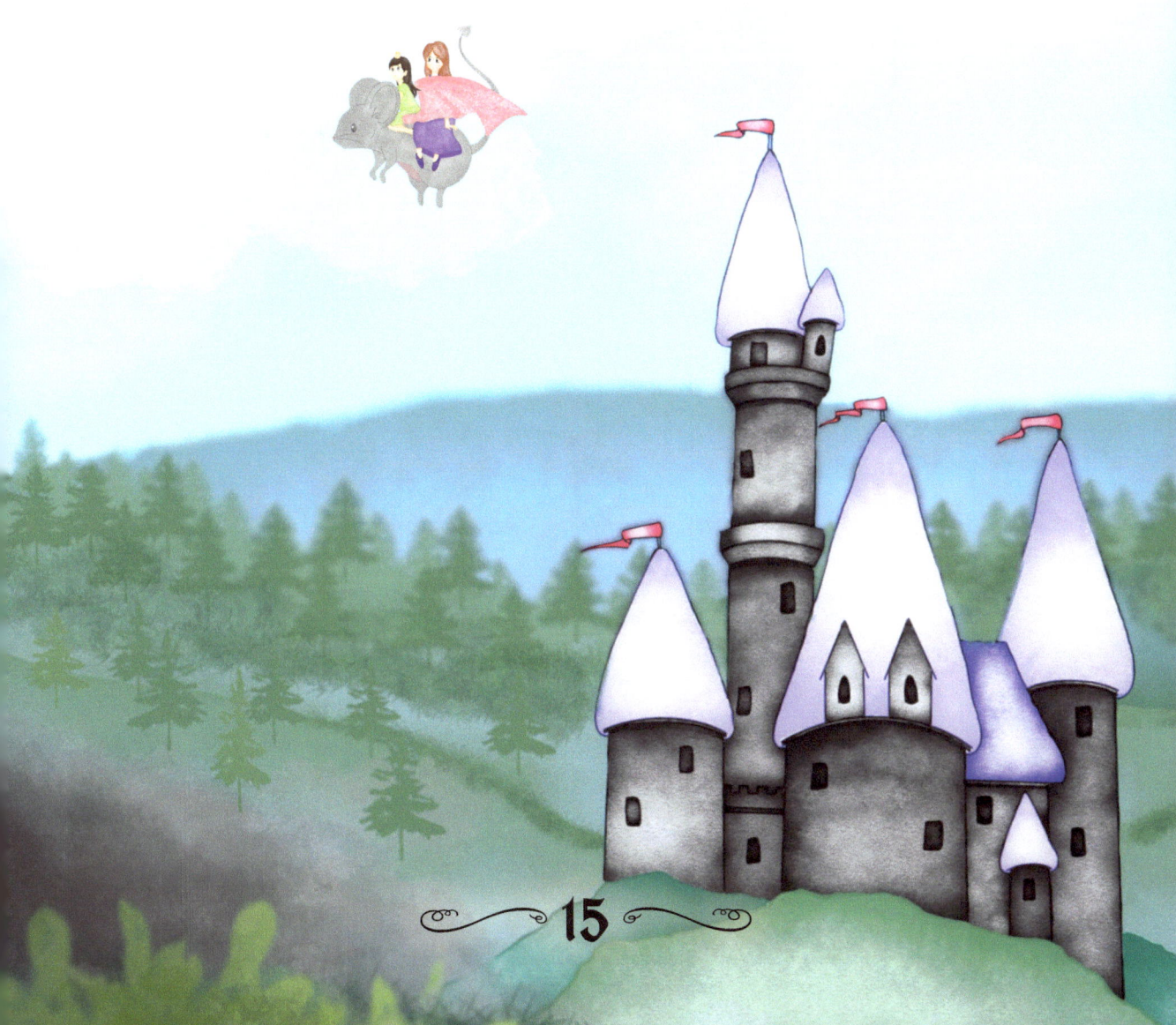

When they landed at the entrance to the Forest of Flowers, they were faced with a thick wall of fog obscuring the path ahead.

"Mama, how are we ever going to find her?" Hannah cried.

"We will find her. We won't stop searching until we–" Elaine stopped suddenly and looked up. "What in the world is that?"

Right above them, a shining orb of light floated lazily through the fog. Within the orb were two tiny moving figures. One figure looked like a much younger Queen Dorothy, and the other was a young child with hair the color of Elaine's. Elaine tried to touch the orb, but her fingers passed through it as if it were nothing but smoke.

"Strange, I don't remember this. Maybe I was too young."

"Mama, what's going on?" Hannah asked.

"I don't know. I don't know why this picture is here or where all this fog came from. Everything seems so dark and dreary! But look at the flowers. They're still so beautiful."

The flowers at their feet were still full of life, glimmering like jewels, while everything else was gray or too far away to see through the dark fog.

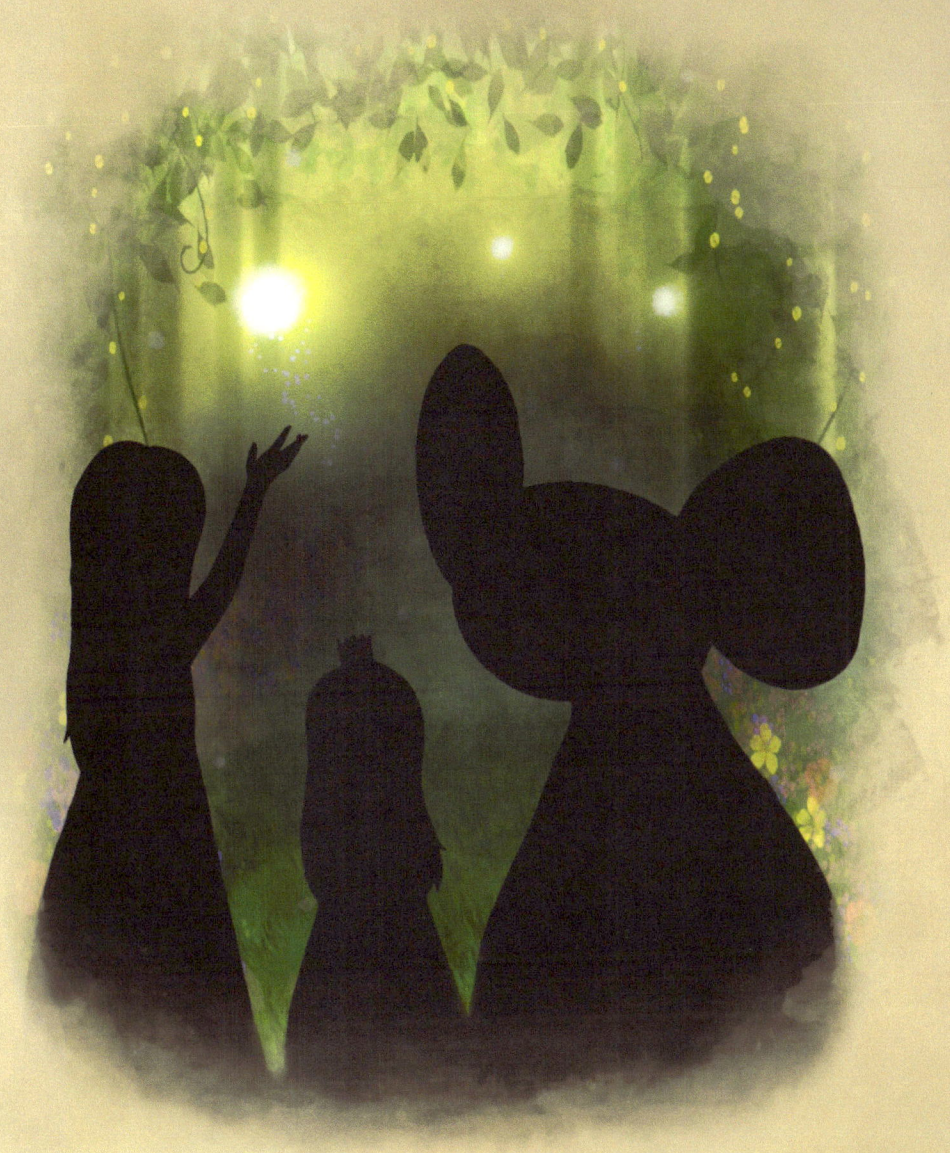

As they looked around, wondering how they'd ever find Queen Dorothy, they could see more images of her floating in the darkness, almost like a picture book.

Chapter Four

Queen Dorothy was very frightened. The fog had gotten so thick she could hardly see, and now she was having trouble breathing, too. *I can't catch my breath! Oh, how will I ever get home? Where is home, anyway?* She knelt on the ground, completely out of breath and starting to panic. She was afraid she might faint.

Just then, she felt a puff of air in her nose and she could breathe again! *What was that?* she thought to herself. Dorothy reached up to her face and felt something long attached to her nose. She held it out in her hands to see what it was. *A vine?* She panicked again and began trying to free herself from it.

As Dorothy fiddled with the vine, she became tangled up and fell to the ground. She pulled with all her might and the vine came off her nose, but she was still in a tangled mess and was having a hard time breathing again.

"Help!" Dorothy cried.

She could see a bright light in the distance but couldn't make out what it was. "Oh, someone please help me!"

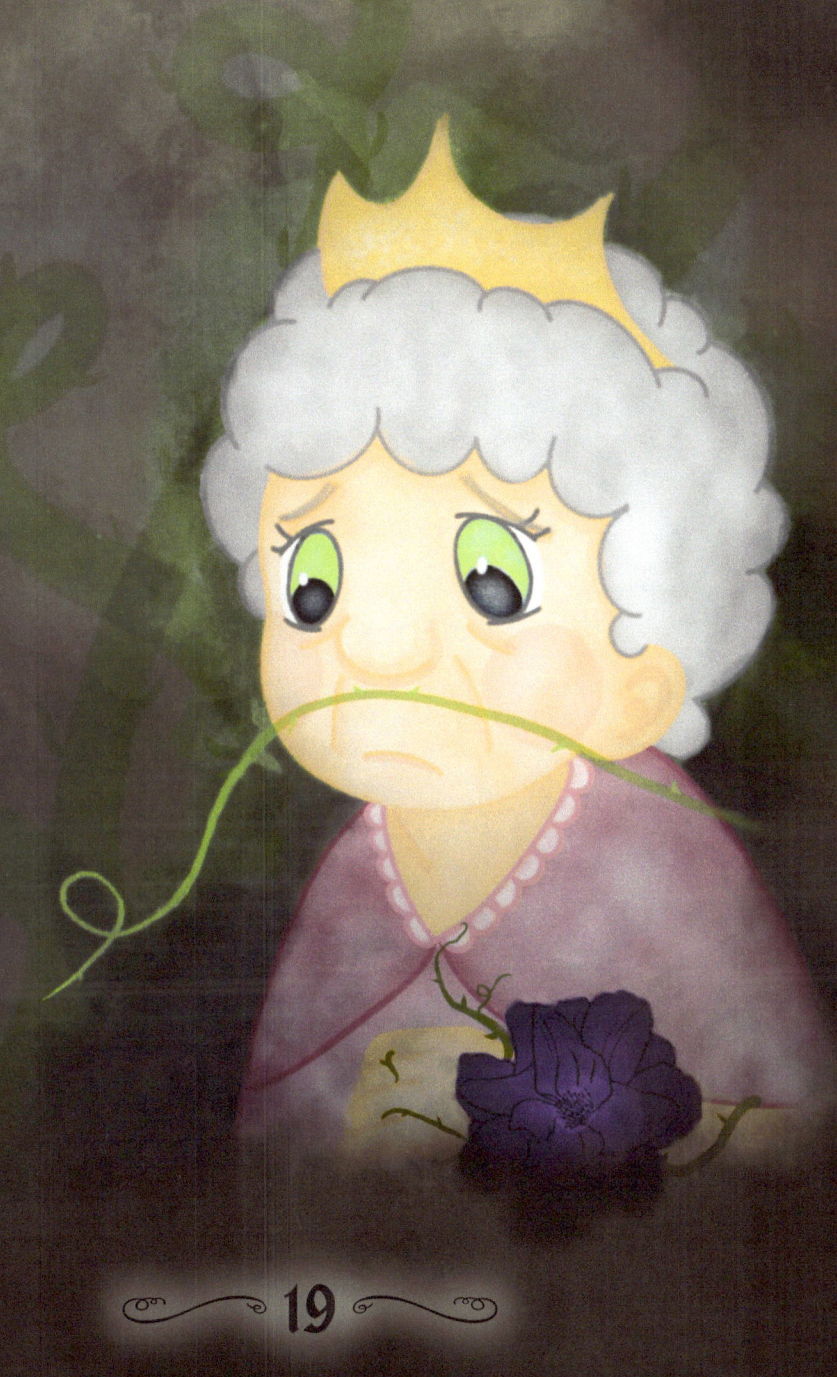

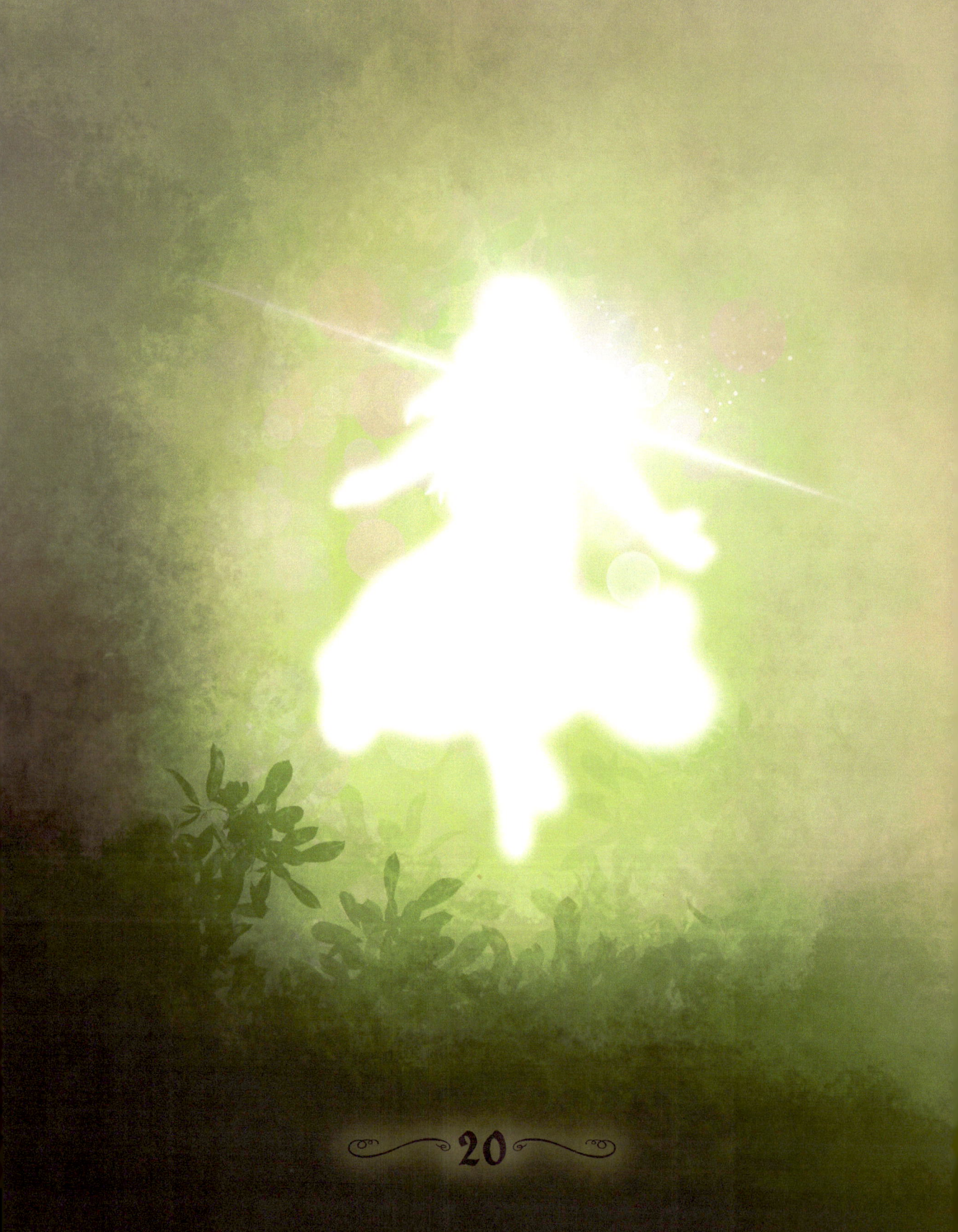

20

The bright, calming light came closer to Dorothy, eventually taking shape. Dorothy looked up with wide eyes; the figure that stood before her looked like a beautiful angel.

"Don't be afraid. I am the Guardian of the Forest of Flowers, caretaker of all who live and grow here. I am here to help you," the Forest Guardian said softly.

"I can't breathe, and I'm all tangled up," Dorothy sobbed.

"It may take a few moments, but just stay calm and I will get you some air."

The Forest Guardian took hold of the vine and began to unwrap it from Dorothy's arms and legs. She then took the end of it and put it up to Dorothy's nose. *Puff!* Dorothy could breathe again!

"Oh, thank you so much!" she exclaimed. "Do you know how I can get home?"

"Where do you live?" the Forest Guardian asked, eyeing the dark purple flower on Dorothy's wrist with apprehension.

"I-I...I don't know. I don't know where I came from. This fog has made me feel very lost and confused." Dorothy realized she didn't remember much of anything anymore.

The Forest Guardian looked away from Dorothy for a moment, staring out into the fog. "I can hear voices in the distance. I will find these people and lead them back here to help you."

"No! Please don't leave me alone! I need my mama and papa!"

The Forest Guardian then held a small bell out to Dorothy. "I have to find help and I must also see for myself how far the Laxness has spread in my forest. Just ring this bell if you need me and I will return to you quickly."

"Okay. Please don't forget about me," Dorothy pleaded.

"I will not forget you. I promise," the Forest Guardian reassured her. Then, she disappeared as quickly as she had come, leaving hazy light hanging in the fog behind her.

Queen Dorothy watched her go and wept softly. *I'm all alone again. I just want my mama and papa! I'm so scared!*

Chapter Five

As Mausdrachen and the two princesses made their way into the forest, Mausdrachen noticed the most beautiful flower he had ever seen. It was purple, sparkling brilliantly even without the sun shining on it.

He felt drawn to the flower and went to smell it.

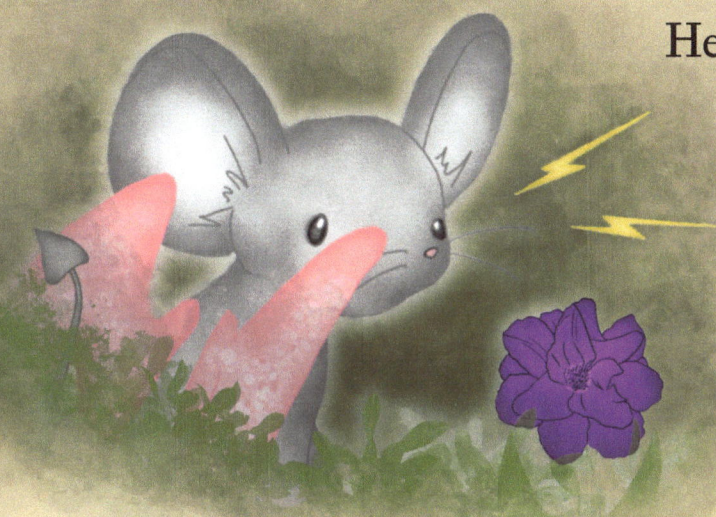

ZZZAAAPPP!!!!

"Squeak!!!" Mausdrachen cried out in pain. Hannah and Elaine hurried to his side.

"Mausy! Are you okay? What happened?"

Mausdrachen rubbed his nose with an enormous paw as Hannah hugged him to comfort him.

"Hannah, look out!" Elaine yelled suddenly. Thorny vines covered with the sparkling purple flowers were rising up behind Hannah, quickly growing toward her hands.

Mausdrachen quickly covered both Elaine and Hannah with his wings, blocking them from the sharp thorns.

ZZZZAAAAAPPPP!!!! One of the flowers zapped him again; he squeaked and jumped. It had hurt, but he was alright.

"Thank you, Mausy! You saved us!" Hannah hugged him again.

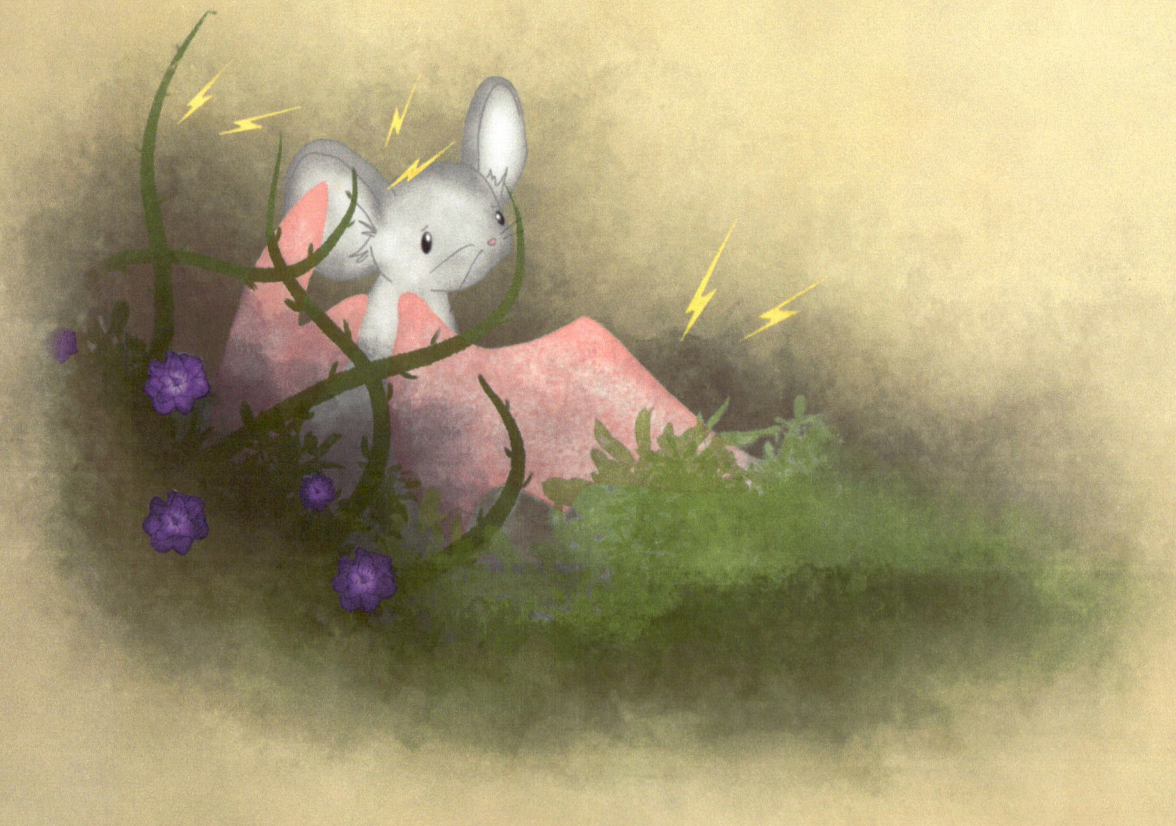

They moved out of reach of the vines, stepping from the path into a clearing in the trees.

Elaine looked up at the fog and gasped. "Hannah! Do you see that?" She pointed at another picture hovering above them.

"Mama, I remember that day! That was when Grandma taught me how to play hide-and-seek!" Hannah replied.

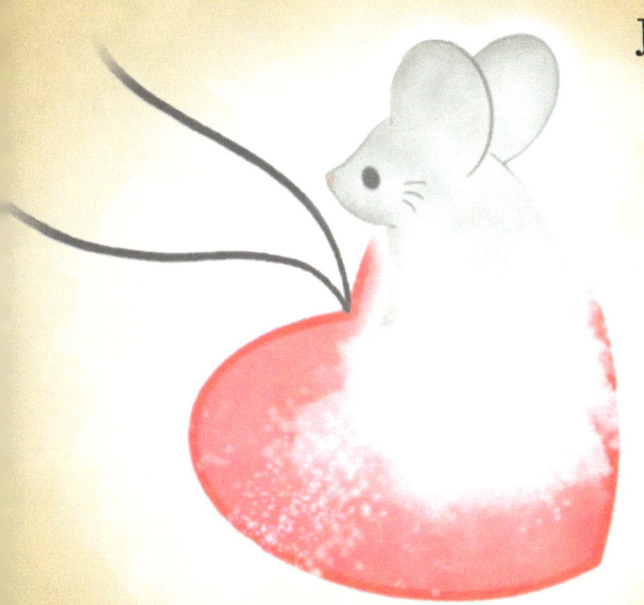

Just then, something came out of the amulet Hannah still wore. It was a mouse made from wisps of light... *It looks like a cute little mouse cloud!* Hannah thought. The little mouse flitted around for a moment before leaping up into the foggy darkness.

The little mouse reached the picture of Hannah playing and grabbed it with its tail, then started floating back down to where Hannah still stood. The picture followed behind the mouse like a kite on a string.

The mouse came all the way back to Hannah before letting go of the picture and immediately disappeared back into the fog. The picture, however, seemed to be pulled closer until it faded into the amulet, which lit up for a moment before dimming again.

"What was that?" Hannah asked, looking back at Mausdrachen and her mother.

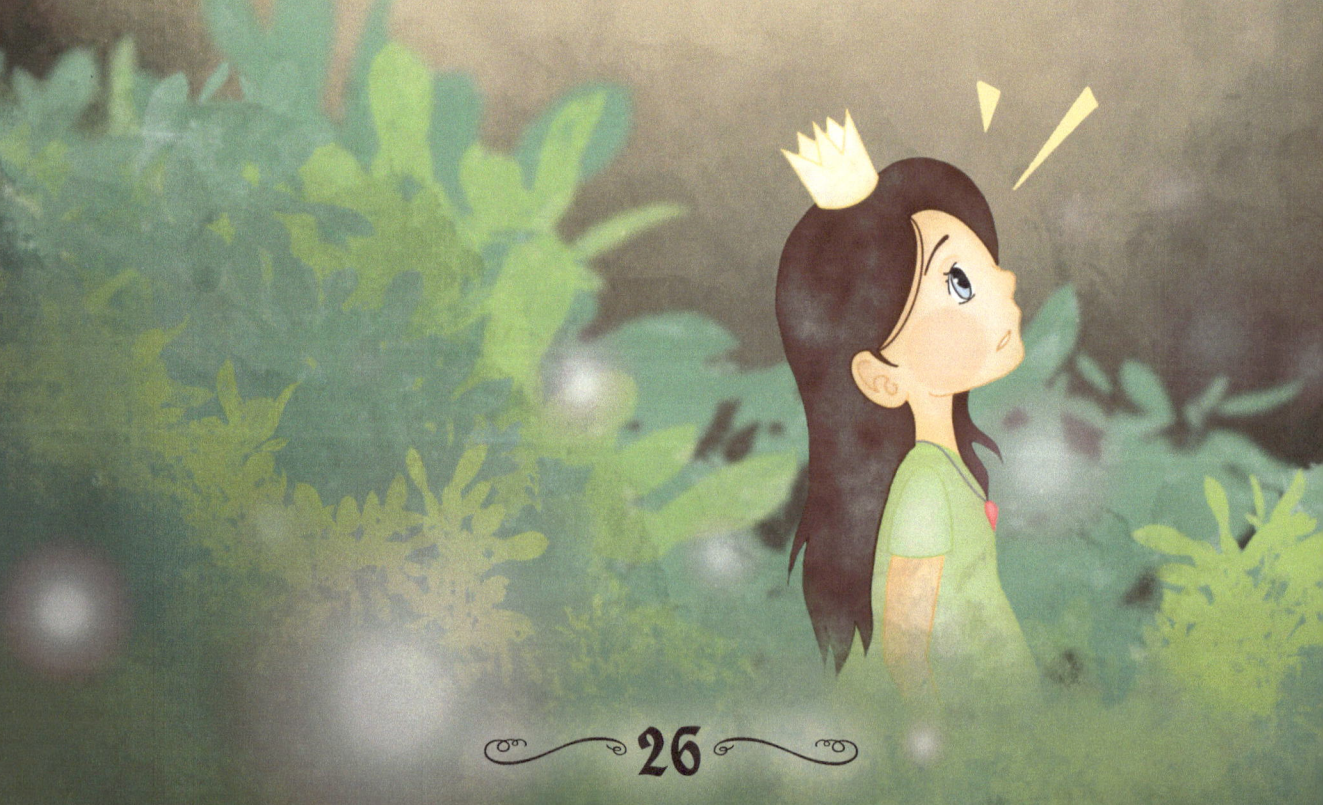

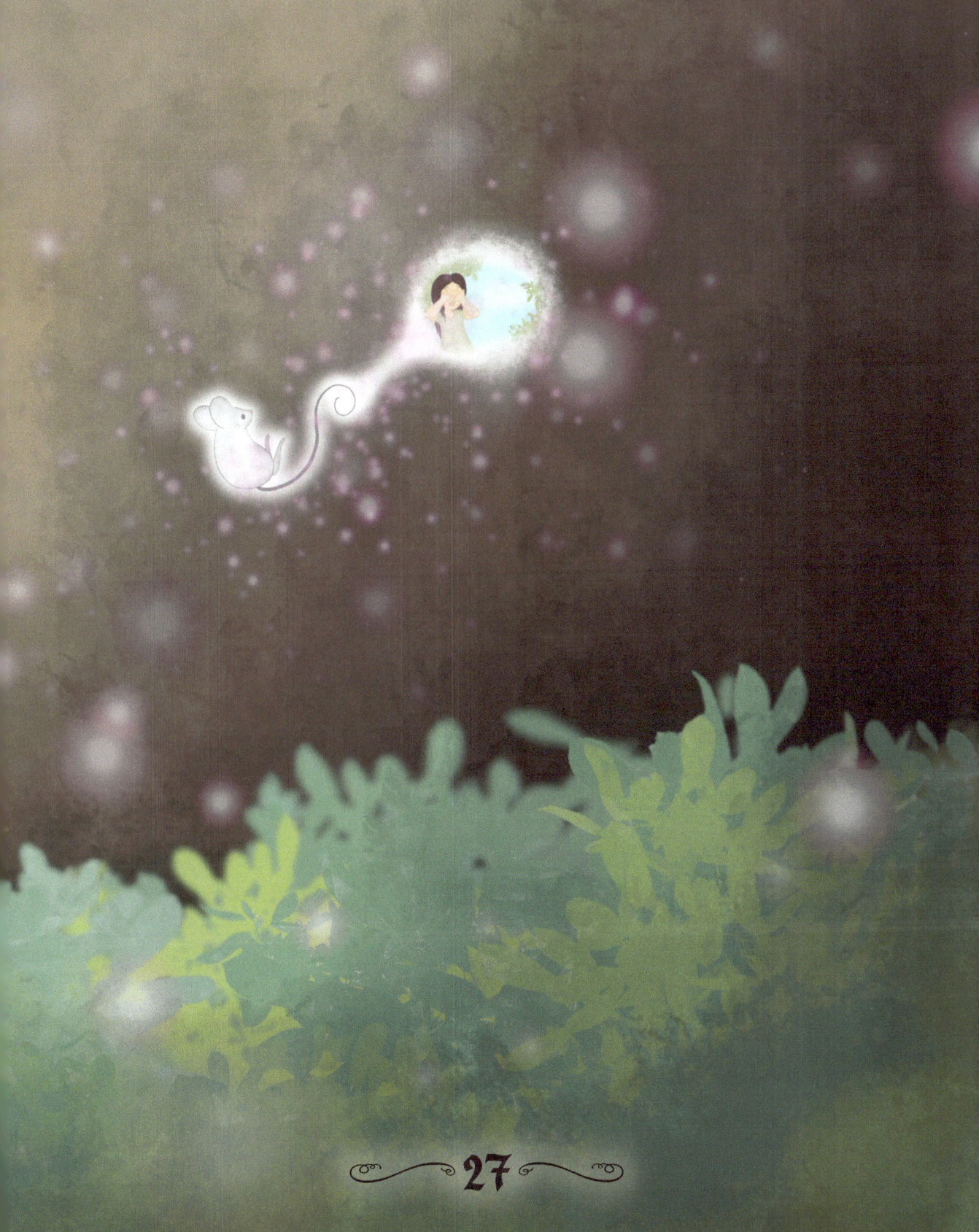

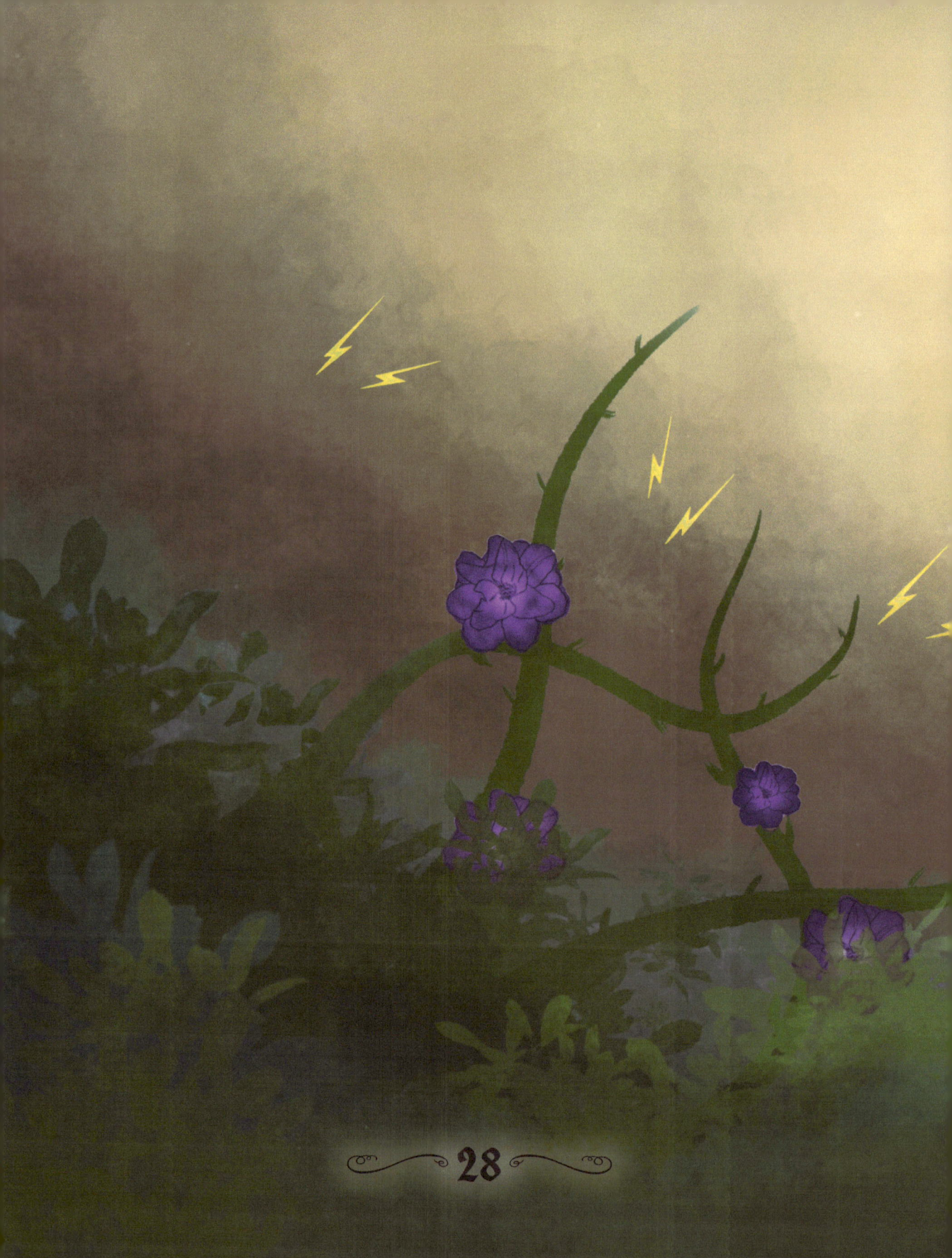

Before Elaine could reply, the purple-flowered vines appeared again, more numerous than before. They were surrounded! The thorns on the vines were long and sharp and the flowers crackled with electricity. They crept closer to Elaine and Hannah, threatening to zap them. Mausdrachen leapt forward and used his wings to protect them as much as he could, but the vines were everywhere.

"Help!" Elaine and Hannah yelled, closing their eyes in fright.

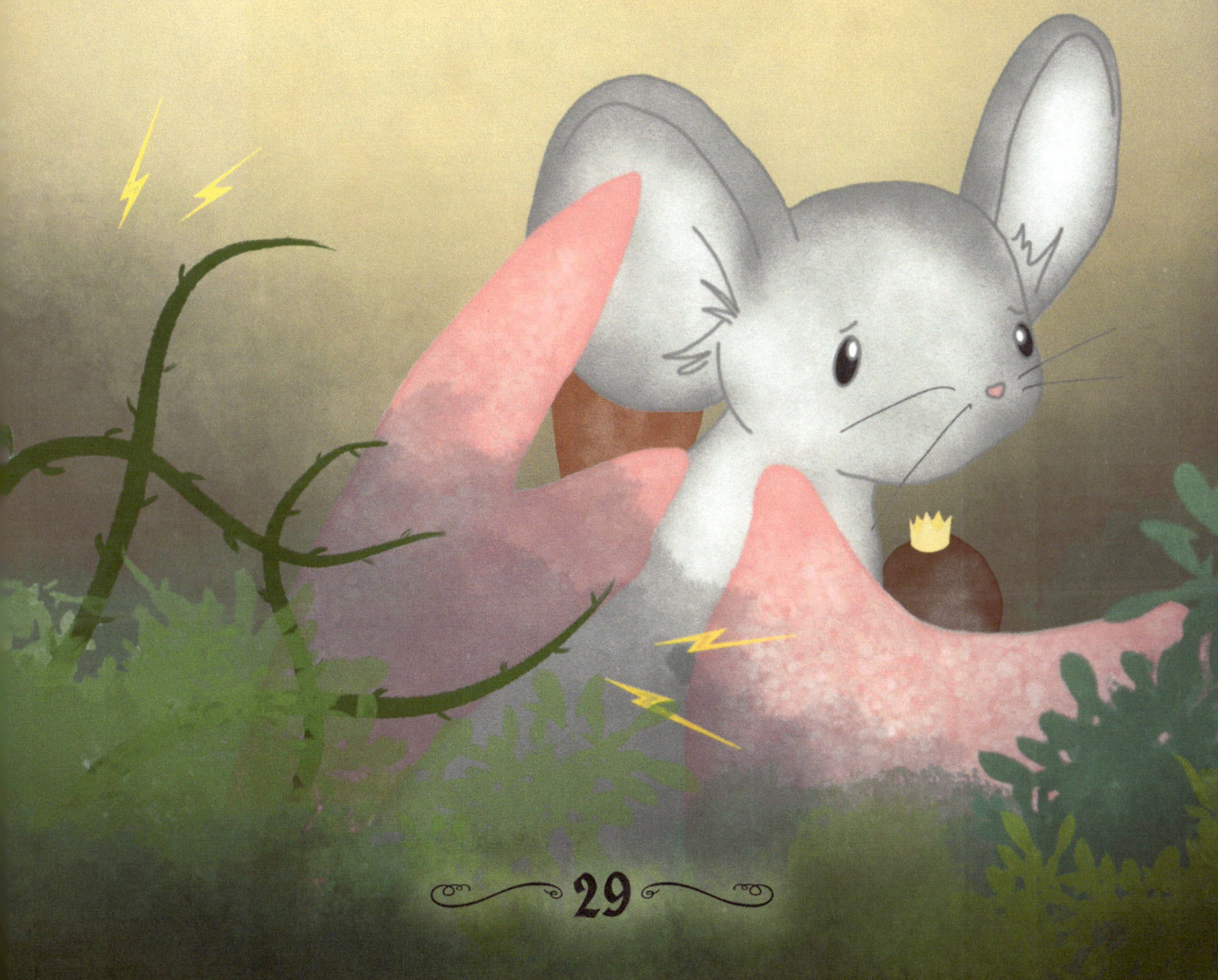

Then, the attacks stopped. They opened their eyes and saw themselves surrounded by a shield of glowing white light. It was such a calming feeling.

"What's happening?" Hannah asked. Mausdrachen and Elaine were silent, their eyes wide as they looked around them

Out of the darkness and fog came an angelic figure. "Greetings, I am the Guardian of the Forest of Flowers. It seems you've found the Laxness."

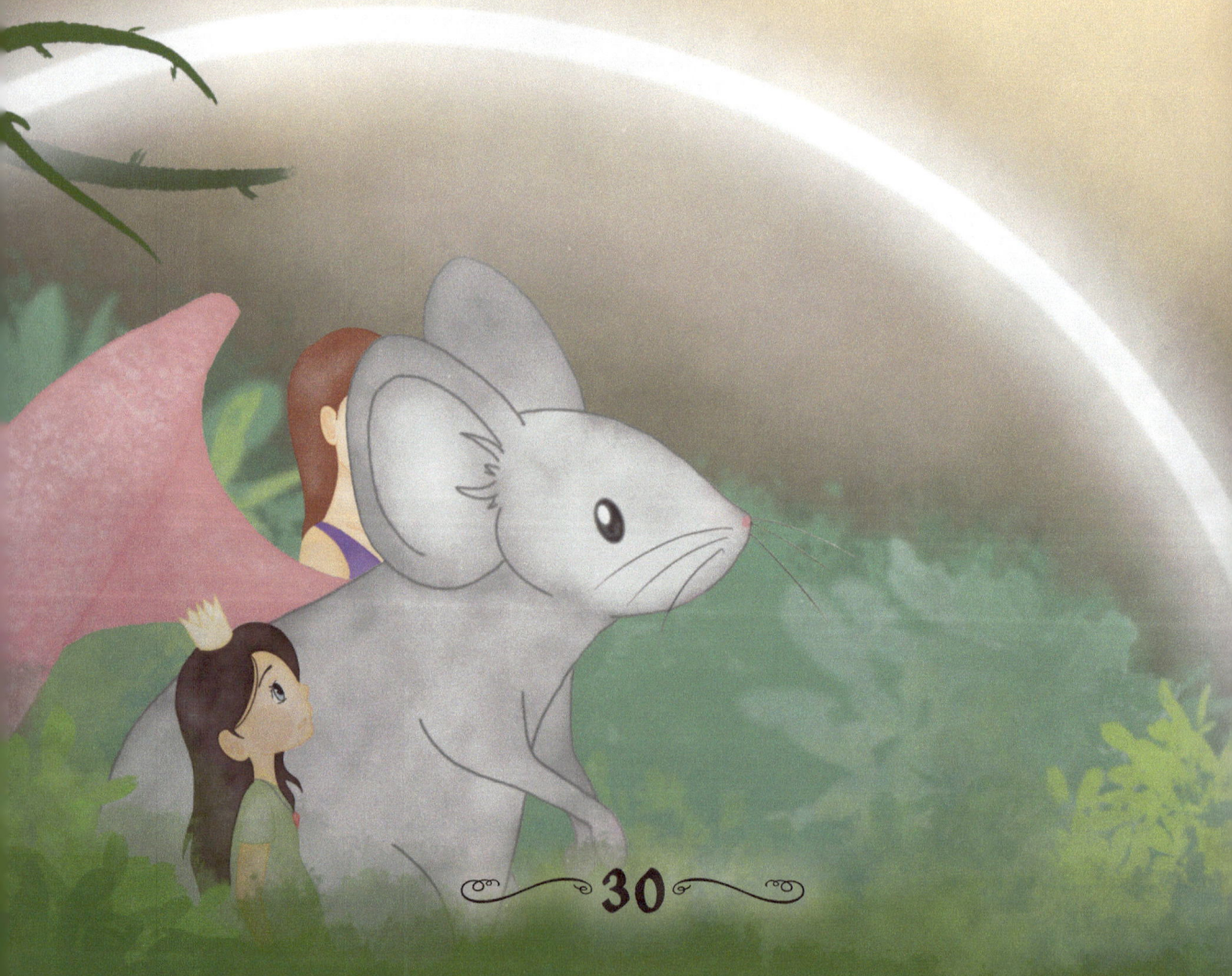

"The Laxness?" Elaine frowned.

"Yes, the Laxness disguises itself as a beautiful flower and feeds on memories. I found a woman here in the forest who has fallen prey to it," the Forest Guardian replied.

"Do you think it could be Grandma?" Hannah asked her mother.

Elaine nodded and turned to the Forest Guardian. "Did she tell you her name? Did she ask for Hannah or Elaine?"

"She only asked for her parents. The Laxness has already taken many of her memories. She looked a lot like this young girl here, only quite a bit older," the Forest Guardian replied, pointing to Hannah.

"That's my grandma!" Hannah exclaimed.

"How are we going to get to her?" asked Elaine.

"I will guide you and keep this shield over you as long as I can, but we need to get your grandmother's memories back to her somehow before it's too late."

Hannah looked down at the heart hanging from a thin silver chain around her neck. "We... We saw a picture of my grandma and me playing hide-and-seek. Then a cloud that looked like a little mouse came out of this amulet and brought the picture to us. The picture went into this amulet and the amulet lit up," Hannah explained, holding up the amulet for the Guardian to see.

"The Queen's amulet? Your grandmother must be the Queen!" the Forest Guardian exclaimed.

She pointed at the amulet, "This is the key to restoring your grandmother's stolen memories. Whenever you remember something special you did with your grandmother, the amulet will collect the memory and keep it safe. The picture that mouse brought you earlier was one of your grandmother's memories. I will guide you to your grandmother, but we must keep trying to recover her memories along the way."

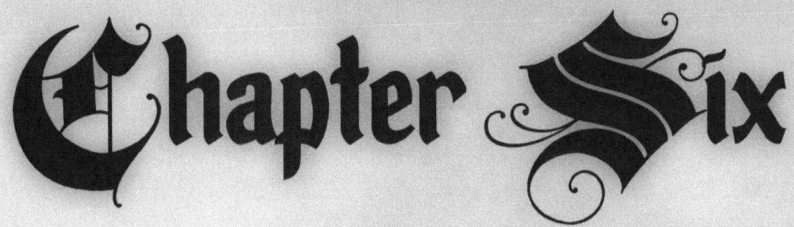

Chapter Six

The Forest Guardian kept the shield over them while they walked down the path. Suddenly, Elaine stopped.

"Hannah, look! There's a picture of you and Grandma dancing in the ballroom over there! Do you remember that day?" she asked, pointing up.

"Yes, it was so much fun! She twirled me all around the ballroom!" Hannah remembered, twirling herself around on the path. She could remember many happy times with her grandmother and it brought a sad smile to her face. *I hope she's okay!*

Suddenly, half a dozen of the wispy little mice escaped from the amulet. All but one charged fearlessly out into the fog, small streaks of light in the darkness. The remaining mouse flew up to fetch the ballroom memory, then started jumping back down to Hannah.

TINK! The mouse bounced off the shield.

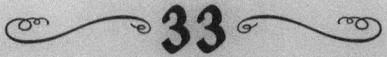

"It would seem my shield is blocking it from getting back in," said the Forest Guardian. "I'll have to open a small part of the shield to let it enter, but beware! As soon as the Laxness sees an opening, it will try to attack again!" The Forest Guardian carefully opened the shield. It was just a small opening at the top, only enough for the mouse to get in, but...

ZAP!

ZAP!

ZAP!

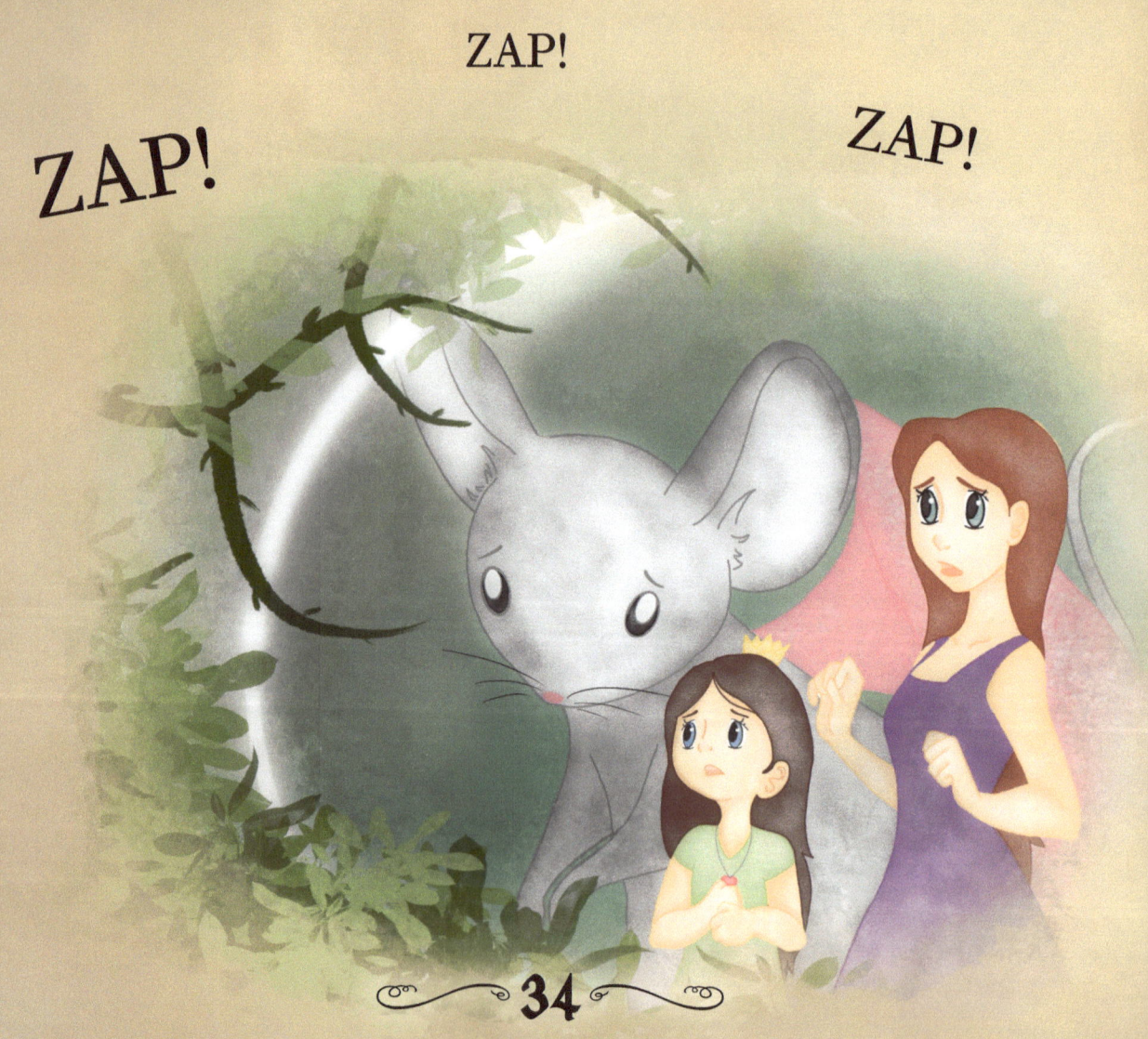

The mouse had come through with the memory, but so had the Laxness' vines. A few were hanging down from the top of the Forest Guardian's shield, sparking and zapping as they reached for the Queen's rescue party.

"SQUEAK!!!" The deadly vines had touched Mausdrachen's outstretched wings.

"Mausy, are you okay?" Hannah asked, scared for her friend.

Mausdrachen's nose still twitched from the shock, but he turned to Hannah and bumped his head gently against hers, letting her know he was okay.

Just then, the rest of the mice from the amulet came flying out of the fog and through the opening in the shield, each with a memory of Dorothy's in tow. They bounded down to where Hannah stood, delivering the memories to the amulet. The amulet grew brighter and brighter with each memory recovered. The mice then leapt back into the fog to recover more of Queen Dorothy's beloved memories.

While the vines above them had been pushed back by the Forest Guardian, and the fog seemed less thick now, the Laxness persisted in its attacks against the shield, hungry for more memories.

Chapter Seven

We should be close to your grandmother now. I can hear her ringing the bell I gave her, and I can see more of the vines that help my forest breathe, too. I had to give one to your grandmother because she was having a hard time breathing on her own," the Forest Guardian explained, pointing down at some delicate light green vines creeping along the ground at their feet.

They passed a large tree and Hannah jumped. "I see her! I see Grandma!" she squealed, pointing up ahead. "Grandma! Grandma!" Hannah ran to her grandmother's side.

"Who are you? I'm not a grandma! Have you seen my mama and papa? I haven't seen them since I went to school today," Dorothy said, then shook the bell the Forest Guardian had given her. "I don't know what this is for, but it makes a pretty sound."

Hannah looked at her mother with tears in her eyes. "What's wrong with Grandma? Why doesn't she know who I am?"

The Forest Guardian looked sad as she explained, "The heart amulet is not full yet. Do you see any more of her memories in the fog?"

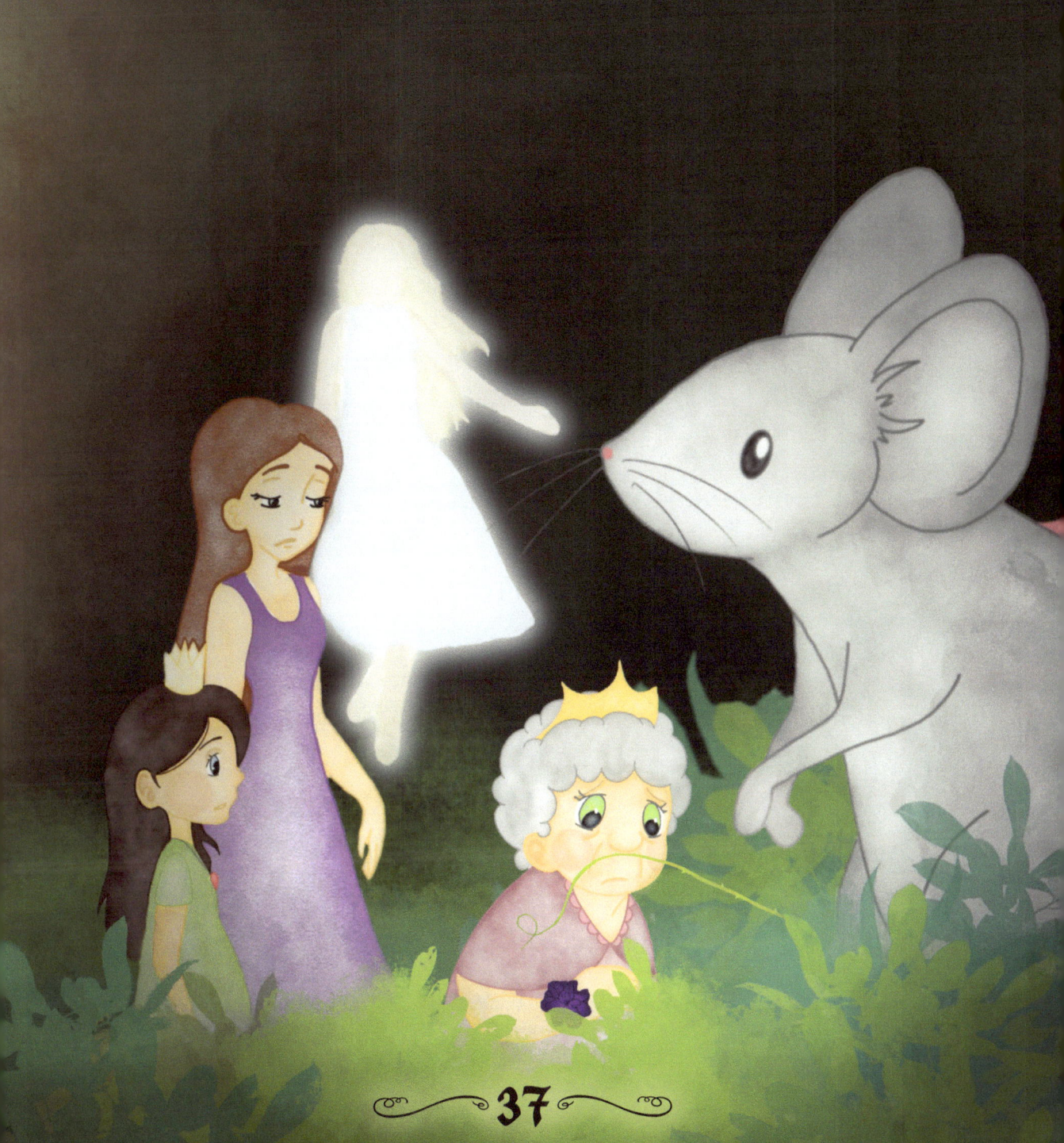

37

They looked all around them for another memory. Finally, Elaine spotted something in the distance. Squinting, she could faintly see another floating ball of light coming toward them. *What memory is that?* she wondered.

As the memory floated closer, Elaine could make out the details. "Hannah, do you see it?" She pointed up, "It's the day you met Mausdrachen! Grandma was holding you and she had a big smile on her face!"

Elaine waited for a minute, expecting a mouse to come jumping out of the fog to collect this last memory, but nothing happened.

"I... I don't remember that," Hannah said, a frown on her face.

Mausdrachen knew what he had to do – how he could help her remember. He turned away from Hannah and launched himself into the air. He began to zigzag and twirl, showing off his best flying tricks. The Laxness vines tried to snag him as he flew past, but Mausdrachen was too quick.

Suddenly, Hannah could remember that day when she'd first met him, when she was a toddler and he was just a young pup. He had been showing off then, too; flying fast through a series of loops, rolls, and dives. Unfortunately, he hadn't been looking where he was going and had crashed into the leafy crown of a tree.

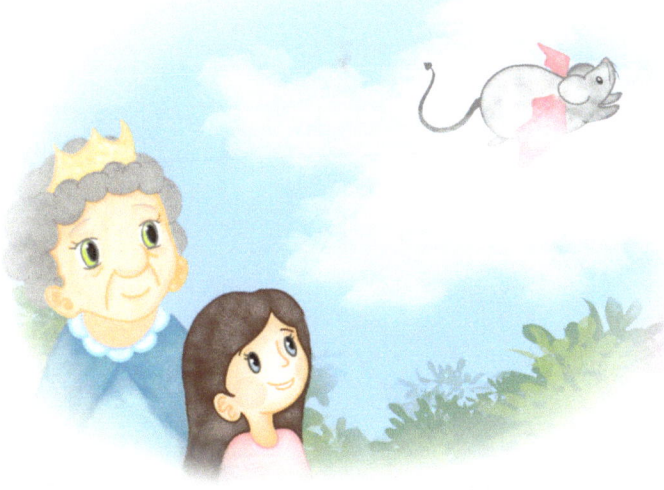

A moment later, he hopped down from the tree, unharmed and only a little embarrassed. Hannah and Dorothy had laughed and clapped for him.

Hannah giggled at the memory. "Mama, I remember now! Mausy was so silly, Grandma and I laughed all the way back to the castle!"

One last little glowing mouse came from the amulet and flew toward the memory as Mausdrachen landed near Hannah. She ran to give him a hug and he nuzzled her hand with his giant whiskery nose.

"Thank you, Mausy. You helped me remember."

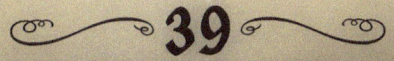

Above them, the last mouse was already coming back with the memory. The Laxness tried to attack it, but failed. The vines were growing weak and the fog was clearing up. The amulet absorbed the last memory and began to glow a beautiful red.

The Forest Guardian came forward then. "The heart is full! Put it on your grandmother. Quickly, child!"

Hannah took the amulet off and carefully put it around her grandma's neck. She watched her grandma's face, waiting for a change, but Dorothy stayed put, looking lost and frightened.

Dorothy peered at them and asked again where they were. "I'm scared," she said quietly.

"It's not working!" Hannah cried, turning back to her mother. "What do we do?"

"Hannah, when you're scared, what does Grandma do to help you?" Elaine asked her, gently smoothing her hair back.

Hannah's face lit up. "She sings!" She turned back to Dorothy and sat down next to her.

"The itsy-bitsy spider went up the waterspout..." Hannah started to sing. She used her hands to do the motions on her grandmother's arm; fingers like a spider walking, and her other hand running down Dorothy's arm to wash the spider away.

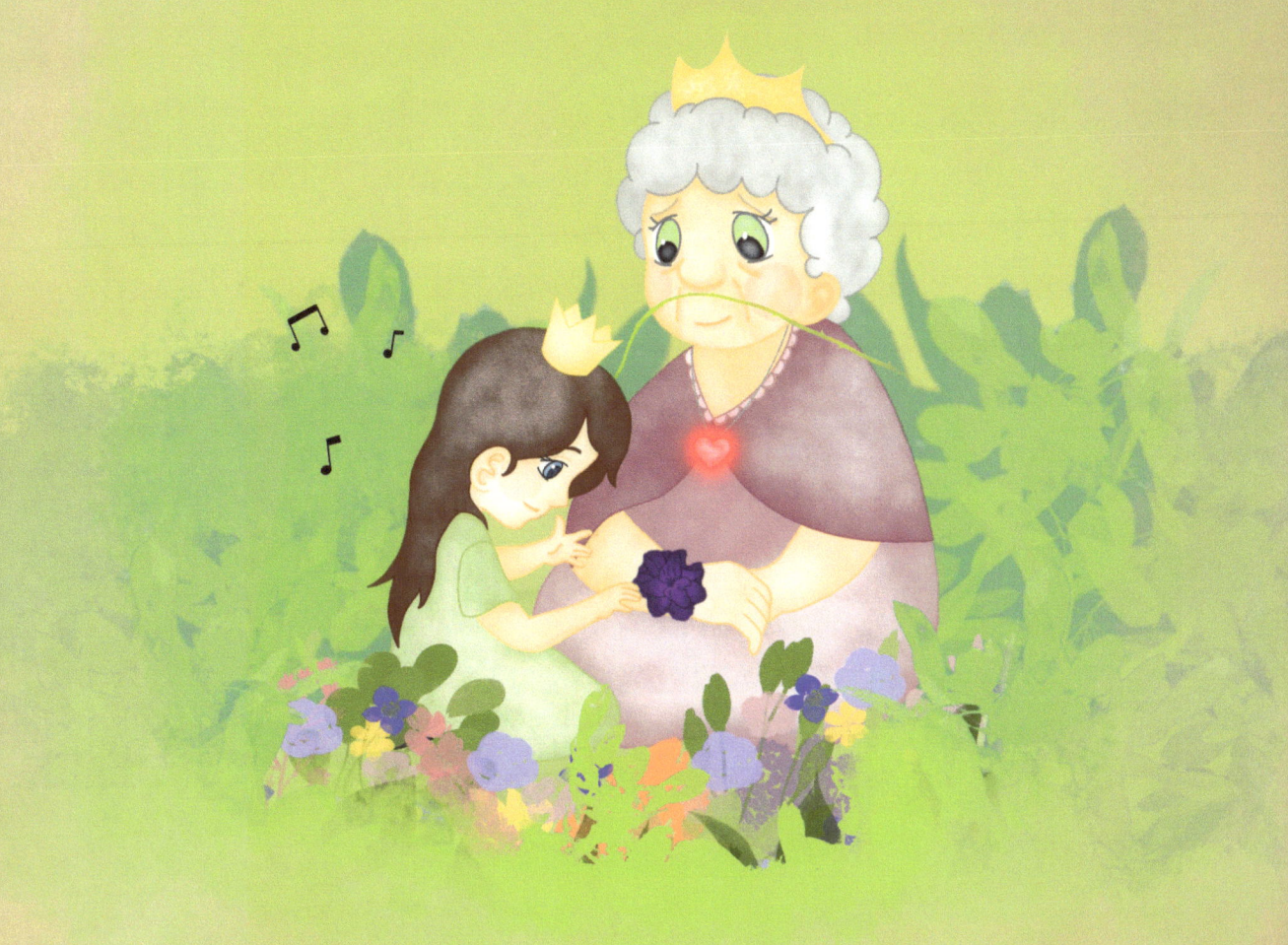

Dorothy laughed and began to sing along. The more they sang, the more Dorothy remembered. By the time they finished singing, Dorothy once again knew where and who she was.

"Hannah, my dear girl!" Queen Dorothy smiled. She hugged Hannah, and Elaine ran to join them. Mausdrachen squeaked with delight, his wings sparkling in the sunshine again now that the fog had gone completely.

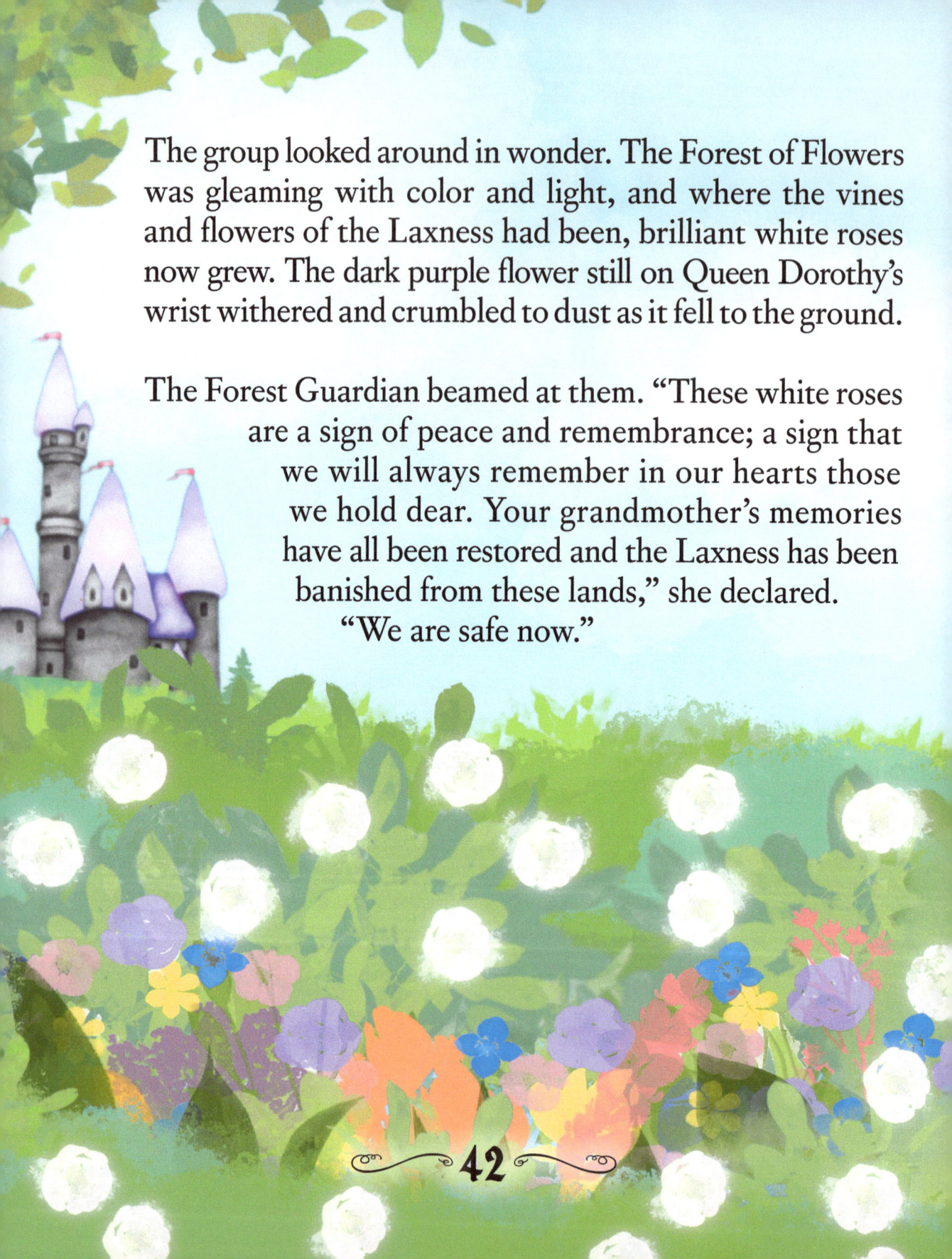

The group looked around in wonder. The Forest of Flowers was gleaming with color and light, and where the vines and flowers of the Laxness had been, brilliant white roses now grew. The dark purple flower still on Queen Dorothy's wrist withered and crumbled to dust as it fell to the ground.

The Forest Guardian beamed at them. "These white roses are a sign of peace and remembrance; a sign that we will always remember in our hearts those we hold dear. Your grandmother's memories have all been restored and the Laxness has been banished from these lands," she declared. "We are safe now."

"So does this mean everything is going to be okay?"
Hannah asked, looking back up at her grandmother.

Queen Dorothy hugged her granddaughter
and daughter close and smiled.
"Yes, my dear Hannah.
Everything is going to
be okay."

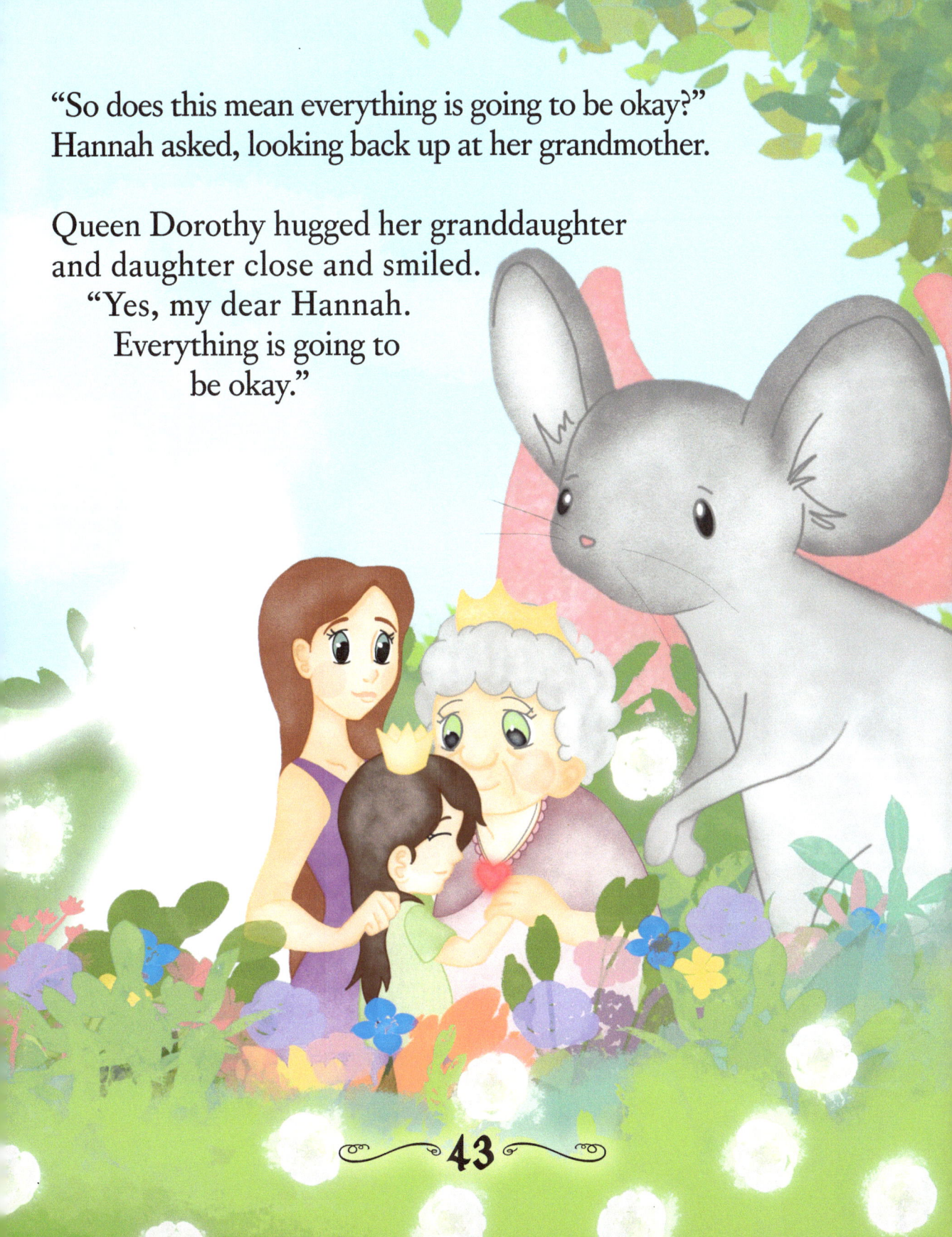

Chapter Eight

Hannah woke up hugging her grandma's favorite stuffed mouse, Mr. Mousey.

What a dream! Oh, I sure do miss Grandma!

She looked out the window at the night sky, and there, floating amongst the clouds, were Grandma and Mausdrachen.

"Grandma, I miss you so much! I wish I could see you more often!"

"You can always visit me in Engelmaus when you dream."

"Okay, Grandma! I'm so glad you're okay now. I'll look after Mama and keep Mr. Mousey safe!"

"I know you will, honey. I'm so proud of you! Now it's your turn to make some memories with Mr. Mousey. Just remember I'm always with you!"

"I will! I love you, Grandma."

"I love you, too, Hannah."

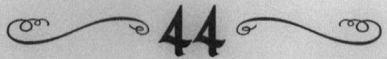

As Mausdrachen and Grandma flew away into the clouds, Hannah looked down at Mr. Mousey and smiled. "Let's go back to sleep, Mr. Mousy. We'll have more adventures first thing tomorrow morning!"

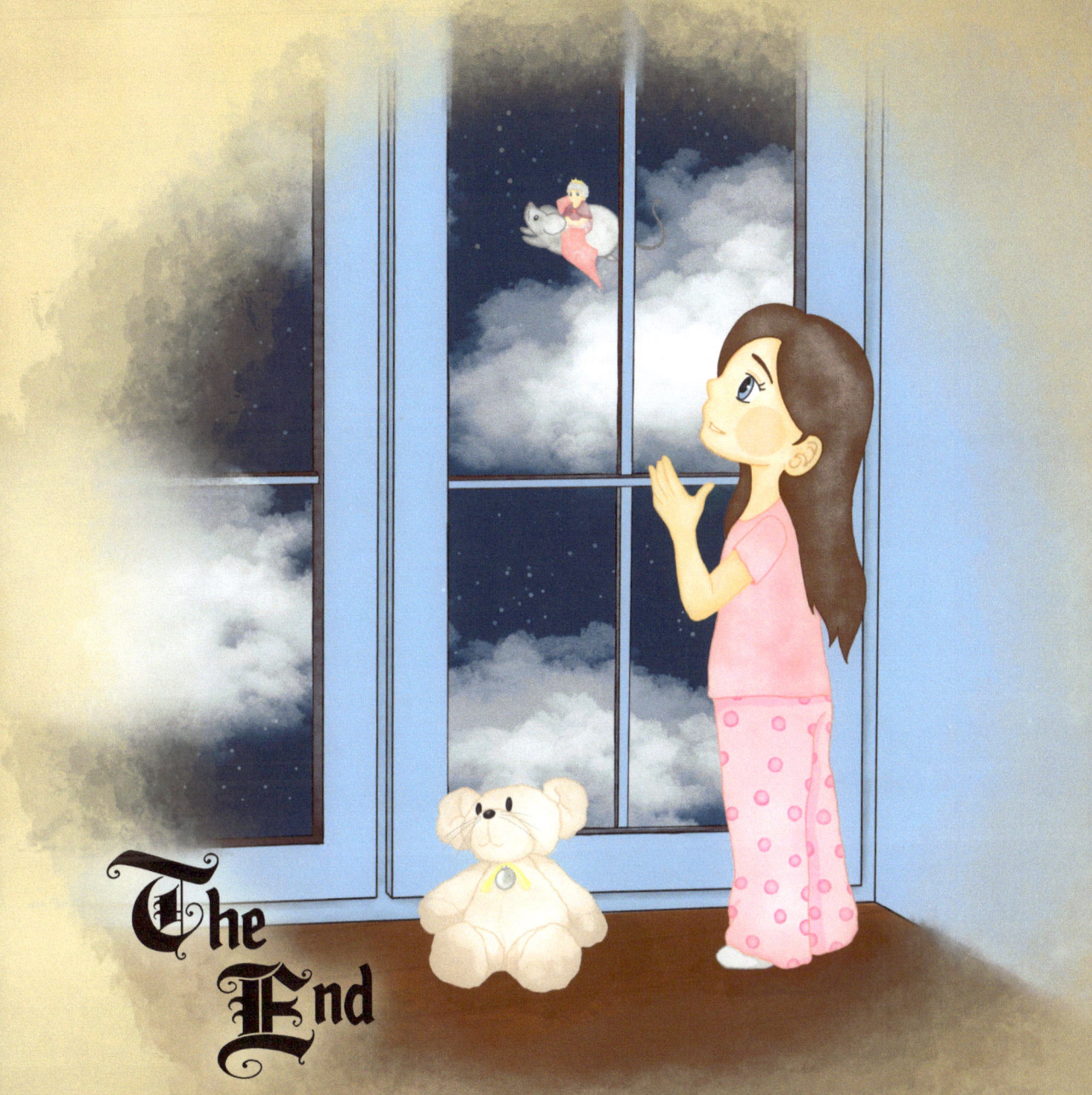

The End

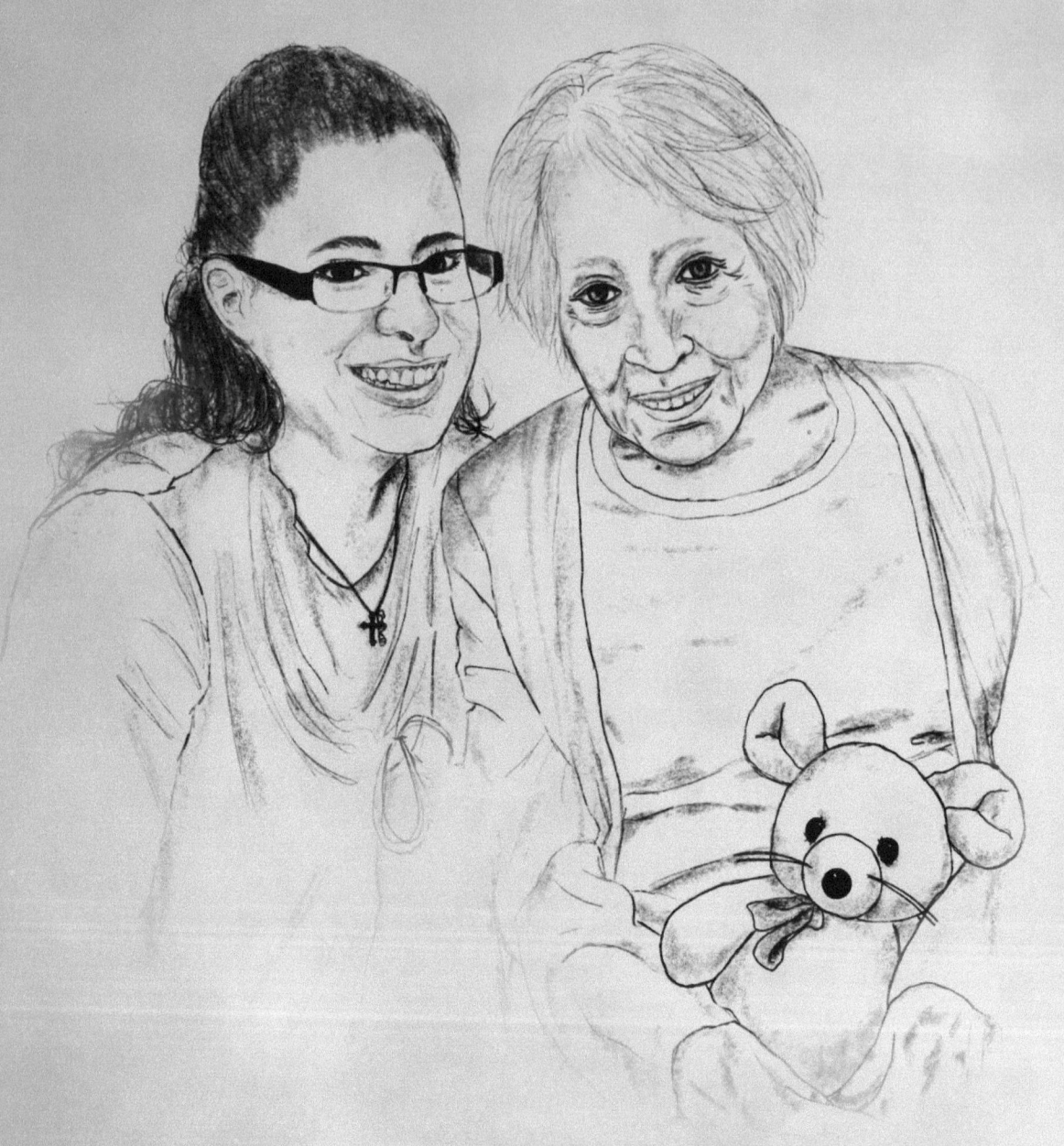

In Memory of Diane Kvamme, 1934–2017

I am at peace now
My memory has been restored
My life was full of adventures
Traveling around the world
I was made of music
As I could play the organ like an angel
My smile lit up a room
My jokes could make anyone happy
I raised a wonderful family
I am proud of every one of them
When my memory faded
Mr. Mousey soothed my fears
I looked back at all I accomplished
And knew it was okay to go
You knew I wasn't broken
Only a little lost for a while
I know you will be sad
But I am no longer suffering
The memories you have of me
Will be cherished forever
One day we will meet again
And I will greet you with open arms
I love you always and forever
I'm your guardian angel now
Watching over you all
See I am not gone
I am always in your heart
When you start to miss me
Just think of me and I'll be there
When you hear music
Know that it is me playing for you
Cherish our precious moments
Until we meet again

Thea Kvamme worked with the elderly for nineteen years before becoming an early-learning teacher. Her mother's diagnoses of and battle with Alzheimer's Disease inspired her to write a book for children to help them understand the changes Alzheimer's can cause in a person.

Thea lives in Minnesota with her four wonderful kids and enjoys writing and knitting. She is currently working on more Mausdrachen books for children.

Samantha Hinton is an artist with a passion for DIY projects and Jurassic Park. *Mausdrachen: Curse of The Laxness* is the first book of her illustration career. She lives in Minnesota with her husband and their two cats, Peanut and Pooper.

Mausdrachen
will return!

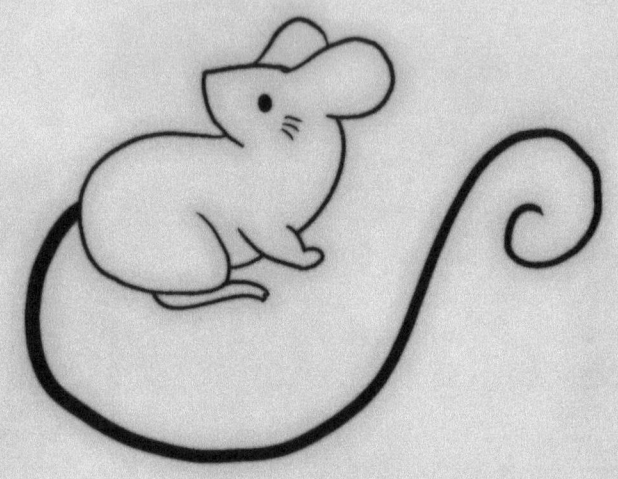

www.ingramcontent.com/pod-product-compliance
Lightning Source LLC
Chambersburg PA
CBHW041618120626
46551CB00003B/486